*The ACR at 75*

# The ACR at 75

## A Diamond Jubilee

Edited by

**David S. Pisetsky MD PhD**

Duke University Medical Center and Durham VA Hospital, Durham, NC

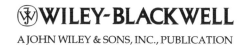

A JOHN WILEY & SONS, INC., PUBLICATION

Published by John Wiley & Sons, Inc., Hoboken, New Jersey
Published simultaneously in Canada

Wiley-Blackwell is an imprint of John Wiley & Sons, formed by merger of Wiley's global Scientific, Technical, and Medical business with Blackwell Publishing.

For general information on our other products and services or for technical support, please contact our Customer Care Department within the United States at (800) 762-2974, outside the United States at (317) 572-3993 or fax (317) 572-4002.

Wiley also publishes its books in a variety of electronic formats. Some content that appears in print may not be available in electronic books. For more information about Wiley products, visit our web site at www.wiley.com.

*Library of Congress Cataloging-in-Publication Data:*

The ACR at 75: A Diamond Jubilee / [edited by] David S. Pisetsky.
        p. ; cm.
    Includes bibliographical references and index.
    ISBN 978-0-470-52377-3 (cloth)
    1.   American College of Rheumatology. 2.   Rheumatology–History. 3.
Arthritis–History.   I.   Pisetsky, David S.   II.   Title: American College of
Rheumatology 75th anniversary reader.
    [DNLM: 1.   American College of Rheumatology. 2.
Rheumatology–history–United States. 3.   Societies, Medical–history–United States.
    4.   Arthritis–history–United States. 5.   Rheumatic
Diseases–history–United States. WE 1 A5126 2009]
    RC927.A78 2009
    616.7'23--dc22                                                              2009011956

Printed in the United States of America.

10 9 8 7 6 5 4 3 2 1

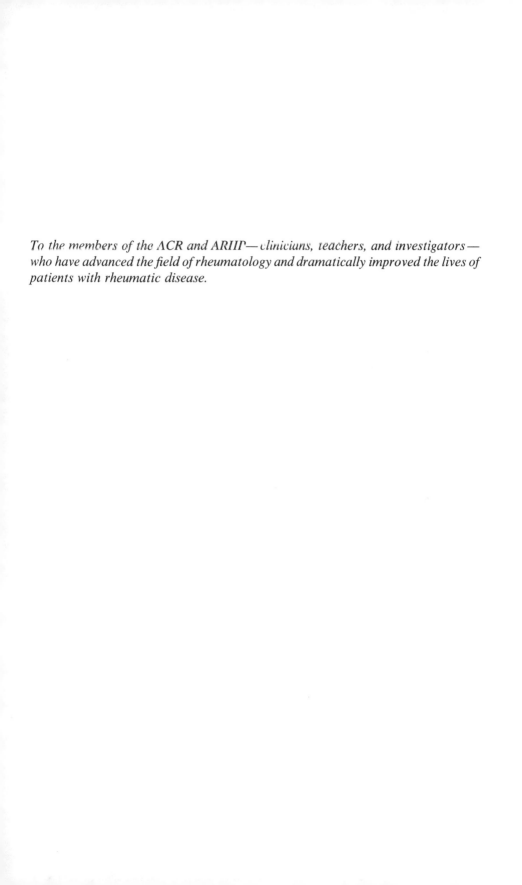

*To the members of the ACR and ARHP—clinicians, teachers, and investigators— who have advanced the field of rheumatology and dramatically improved the lives of patients with rheumatic disease.*

# Contents

# *Preface*

In 2009, the American College of Rheumatology (ACR) commemorates its diamond jubilee, celebrating 75 years of remarkable accomplishment. An important reason for a diamond jubilee's special quality derives from the scale of human life. A person who turns 75 has happily gone beyond the Biblical three score and ten, and a marriage or monarchy of 75 years is as rare as it is momentous. Although an organization at 75 years is just getting started, the allusion to a person is too strong and compelling to resist.

For the ACR, the clan and well wishers will assemble in Philadelphia for the party, and any celebration of this magnitude needs an anniversary album to savor the past. This volume is that album, and it is filled with goodies, including recollections, reminiscences, history, speculation, reflection, contemplation, and wonderful science. Like all good birthday albums, there are baby pictures. Rather than the cute images of junior as a toddler, the ACR baby shots are fuzzy images of serious men in suits captured in black and white and labeled no doubt with a fountain pen because Magic Markers did not exist then.

Looking back to the founding of the ACR and its predecessor, the American Rheumatism Association (ARA), inspires admiration and awe for those present at the creation. Times then were tough. The world was deep into a depression that dwarfs today's economic downtown in size and psychological impact. The world was also edging toward a cataclysmic war. In medicine, times were also tough. Therapy was primitive, relying on drugs that were dangerous, unproven, or ineffective. In the absence of established treatments for rheumatic disease, the job of a rheumatologist was to watch by almost helplessly as disease progressed relentlessly to severe disability and early death.

Nevertheless, the founders of the ACR had faith in the prospects for a better world for patients and established an organization that has propelled rheumatology to where it is today. For the Association of the Rheumatology Health Professionals (ARHP), the path was perhaps more complicated given its disparate membership and affiliation with the Arthritis Foundation, but this section of today's ACR has a unique role. In its focus on interdisciplinary care, outcomes research, and quality of life, the ARHP has made rheumatology a leader in the care of patients with chronic disease and the importance of patient concerns in determining the efficacy of therapy.

Whereas the success of the ACR is evident using many metrics—membership, meeting attendance, impact factor of *Arthritis & Rheumatism*, and research funding through the Research and Education Foundation (REF)—the overriding value is truly its impact on the lives of patients with rheumatic disease. There is no question that the treatment of virtually every major rheumatic disease has improved dramatically in the past decades in the way that ACR founders could never have imagined, even if they were as futurist in their thinking as Jules Verne. In the 1930s, neither antibodies nor cytokines were known, and the idea of anticytokine therapy to treat rheumatoid arthritis could not have been even fantasized. Verne knew the moon was there and a space ship is not that far away in concept from a train, especially because he knew from fireworks that a rocket could propel objects into the sky.

This preface is just a beginning, and I want to extend a welcome to readers to enjoy marvelous essays contained in this volume. In my invitation letter to authors, I asked them to be interesting, engaging, and personal. They have fulfilled this request admirably, and I want to thank them for their great writing in recounting the story of the ACR, ARHP, and REF from past to present; they have even provided a look in the future. I also want to thank Rachel Myslinski and Naami Davidai on the staff of the ACR for their yeoman work in communicating with authors and for their great assistance with assembling this volume.

Although the success of the ACR derives from the energy and commitment of its members, keeping rheumatology moving forward requires a wide array of professional skills beyond the purview of health care providers. Since its establishment as an independent organization, the ACR has had outstanding staff in Atlanta. These individuals have been extraordinary in their activities and have worked tirelessly to optimize the work of the volunteers of ACR and ARHP. Currently, the ACR office has 70 staff and oversees an organization of 8000 members and a yearly budget of $18 million. The staff also coordinates an international meeting that grows each year in size and scope; today, this meeting fills conventional halls that stretch a mile in length. The first meeting of the ARA had 75 attendees, which could barely fill a ballroom in a small hotel.

Over the years, I have been privileged and fortunate to work with many talented and devoted staff members of the ACR. These people are all consummate professionals who can negotiate the complexity of running a large organization whose members have full-time jobs and are busy taking care of patients or doing research. I can name tens of staff whose work merits commendation, but I will restrict myself to a very few. Space limits those I can name, but on behalf of ACR members past and present, I extend my kudos and appreciation to you all.

As the Executive Vice President, Mark Andrejeski is a superb administrator who combines a deep commitment to rheumatology with keen business acumen and organizational skill. Mark has served with great distinction since the ACR became independent and has done a tremendous job as the organization has grown and diversified. Lynn Bonifglio, who is a Master of the ACR, worked for the organization for 51 years. She brought warmth, joy, and good spirit to everything she did and treated the ACR like family. In her years as the director of membership, she derived great happiness not just for the success of the ACR but from the accomplishment of each and every member. Jane Diamond, Senior Director and Managing Editor, has an appropriate name. She wants *Arthritis & Rheumatism* to be a jewel, and in her care and attention to detail, she is like a diamond cutter who must get it right. Finally, Ron Olejko, senior director of the annual meeting, is an animating spirit and impresario of the world's finest medical meeting. Ron wants everyone to have a great time wherever the meeting occurs, and he orchestrates this complex undertaking with ebullience and aplomb. As they say at the Academy Awards, there is not enough time to thank everyone who made this happen.

I will save my last acknowledgments for the volunteers and leaders of the ACR, ARHP, and REF who, as they say in current lingo, have taken time out from their busy schedules to work for the organization. Through their service on committees, task forces, and review panels, the volunteers keep the ACR running in high gear and have developed innovative, high-quality programs to meet the needs of the times. Among these individuals, the presidents of the organizations have done spectacular work and have led with great vision and intelligence. Delivering clinical care, administrating a division or department, or conducting research is a huge undertaking by itself. Add to that committee work, extensive travel, conference calls, fundraising, lobbying, press conferences, and now 24/7 responsiveness to e-mails from members and that work becomes gigantic. Nevertheless, the presidents have given greatly of themselves and have assured that mission of the ACR is accomplished. At the party in Philadelphia, we will toast you all.

The chapters in this book tell a great story. To everyone, Happy Anniversary, congratulations, keep up the good work, and best of luck for the future.

DAVID S. PISETSKY

# *Contributors*

STEVEN B. ABRAMSON, MD, Hospital for Joint Diseases/NYU, Department of Rheumatology/Medicine, New York, NY

NEAL S. BIRNBAUM, MD, Pacific Rheumatology Association, San Francisco, CA

DAVID G. BORENSTEIN, MD, Arthritis & Rheumatism Associates, Washington, DC

DENNIS W. BOULWARE, MD, Kaiser Permanente Medical Center, Honolulu, HI

TERESA J. BRADY, PhD, Center for Disease Control, Arthritis Program, Atlanta, GA

FERDINAND C. BREEDVELD, Leiden University Medical School, Leiden, the Netherlands

GERD-RÜDIGER BURMESTER, Department of Rheumatology and Clinical Immunology, Charité–University Medicine Berlin, Berlin, Germany

JAMES T. CASSIDY, MD, University of Missouri HSC, Department of Child Health, Columbia, MO

ANTONIO LA CAVA, UCLA School of Medicine, Rehabilitation Center, Los Angeles, CA

CHARLES L. CHRISTIAN, MD, University of Florida School of Medicine, Gainesville, FL

LESLIE J. CROFFORD, MD, University of Kentucky, Division of Rheumatology, Lexington, KY

MAXIME DOUGADOS, Department of Rheumatology, Cochin Hospital Medical Faculty, Descartes University, Paris, France

PAUL EMERY, MD, Chapel Allerton Hospital, Academic Unit of Musculoskeletal Disease, Leeds, England

EPHRAIM P. ENGLEMAN, MD, University of California Medical School, San Francisco, CA

MARC FELDMANN, PhD, Kennedy Institute of Rheumatology, Cytokine Biology and Immunology, London, UK

DAVID T. FELSON, MD, Boston University School of Medicine, Clinical/Research Training Unit, Boston, MA

DAVID A FOX, Division of Rheumatology, Department of Internal Medicine, University of Michigan, Ann Arbor, MI

SHERINE E. GABRIEL, MD, Health Sciences Research, Mayo Clinic, Rochester, MN

MARY B. GOLDRING, Hospital for Special Surgery, New York, NY

STEVEN R. GOLDRING, MD, Hospital for Special Surgery, New York, NY

PETER K. GREGERSEN, MD, Feinstein Institute Medical Research, Genomics and Human Genetics, Manhasset, NY

BEVRA H. HAN, MD, UCLA School of Medicine, Rehabilitation Center, Los Angeles, CA

EDWARD D. HARRIS, JR., MD, Alpha Omega Alpha, Menlo Park, CA

TOM W.J. HUIZINGA, Department of Rheumatology, Leiden University Medical Center, Leiden, The Netherlands

JEFFREY N. KATZ, MD, Brigham and Women's Hospital, Rheumatology, Boston, MA

JONATHAN KAY, MD, University of Massachusetts Medical School, Worcester, MA

WILLIAM N. KELLEY, MD, University of Pennsylvania School of Medicine, Rheumatology Division, Philadelphia, PA

LARS KLARESKOG, MD, PhD, Karolinska University Hospital, Rheumatology Unit, Stockholm, Sweden

MICHAEL D. LOCKSHIN, MD, Hospital for Special Surgery-Cornell, New York, NY

MARIAN A. MINOR, PhD, University of Missouri, Physical Therapy, Columbia, MO

RAVINDER NATH MAINI, Kennedy Institute of Rheumatology, Imperial College School of Medicine, Hammersmith, London, England

JAMES R. O'DELL, MD, University of Nebraska Medical Center, Department of Internal Medicine, Nebraska Medical Center, Omaha, NE

RICHARD S. PANUSH, MD, Saint Barnabas Medical Center, Department of Medicine, Livingston, NJ

DAVID S. PISETSKY, MD, PhD, Duke University Medical Center and Durham VA Hospital, Durham, NC

H. RALPH SCHUMACHER, JR., MD, VA Medical Center, Philadelphia, PA

RAM PYARE SINGH, UCLA School of Medicine, Rehabilitation Center, Los Angeles, CA

RAM RAJ SINGH, UCLA School of Medicine, Rehabilitation Center, Los Angeles, CA

BRIAN SKAGGS, UCLA School of Medicine, Rehabilitation Center, Los Angeles, CA

JOSEF S. SMOLEN, MD, Krankenhaus Lainz, 2nd Department of Medicine, Vienna, Austria

ENG M. TAN, MD, Scripps Research Institute, W M Keck Autoimmune Disease Center, La Jolla, CA

BETTY P. TSAO, UCLA School of Medicine, Rehabilitation Center, Los Angeles, CA

MICHAEL E. WEINBLATT, MD, Brigham and Women's Hospital, Rheumatology and Immunology, Boston, MA

GERALD WEISSMANN, MD, New York University Medical Center, Department of Medicine, New York, NY

MAIDA WONG, UCLA School of Medicine, Rehabilitation Center, Los Angeles, CA

EDWARD H. YELIN, PhD, Arthritis Research Group, University of California, San Francisco, CA

# Chapter 1

# The History of ACR: Before 1970

**Ephraim P. Engleman**

*University of California Medical School, San Francisco, CA*

If it was rheumatism, then there had to be a focus of infection [1]. And so, teeth were extracted, as were tonsils, or gall bladders, or any other easily accessible organs. And if that technique did not succeed, there was always the autogenous vaccine (later refuted [2]). Finally, how about a high colonic irrigation to "rid the body of toxic wastes" [3]? That is the way it was in the United States less than 100 years ago.

The Europeans saw the light ahead of us [3,4]. By 1925, with the leadership of the Dutch physician Jan van Bremen, interested physicians of several European countries agreed to collaborate in the study and control of rheumatic diseases. In 1926, Louis B. Wilson, Director of the Mayo Foundation for Medical Education and Research, visited van Bremen. Dr. Wilson was so impressed by van Bremen's efforts that he immediately reported them to many of his American colleagues. What followed 2 years later was the 15-member American Committee for the Control of Rheumatism

*The ACR at 75: A Diamond Jubilee*
Copyright © 2009 by John Wiley & Sons, Inc.

(ACCR), chaired by Ralph Pemberton of Philadelphia.* Dr. Pemberton's interest in arthritis had been stimulated by his observations of soldiers with arthritis during WW I [5].

From the very beginning of discussions by the ACCR, and with the enthusiastic endorsement of the eminent orthopedist Robert Osgood of Boston, it was agreed that the fight against rheumatism belonged in the category of internal medicine, and no other discipline could properly launch such a broad effort. An editorial in the *Journal of the American Medical Association (JAMA)* written by Pemberton, stated the purposes of ACCR: "to stimulate professional and lay interest in arthritis, research and education, the development of a nomenclature and to publicize therapeutic measures of proven value" [6].

An early and difficult task of the ACCR was nomenclature and classification of rheumatic diseases. Undertaken by a subcommittee chaired by Russell Cecil of New York and later by Walter Bauer of Boston, it was agreed that the pathologic distinctions between inflammatory and noninflammatory joint disease, as demonstrated by Nichols and Richardson, should be the basis of their deliberations [7]. It was not until 1941 that a "provisional classification" was actually adopted [8].

The first annual, open scientific meeting of the ACCR was held in New Orleans in 1932 [9]. Chaired by Dr. Pemberton, it was a 3-hour session in which 11 papers were read and discussed (see Figure 1.1).† Two years later, the Committee became an Association, The American Association for the Study and Control of Rheumatic Diseases [4]. The goals of the Association were similar to those of the Committee. It would be limited "to approximately 100 members including physicians and laymen with interest in public health and medical administration."

At an undetermined time after the creation of the American Association for the Study and Control of Rheumatic Diseases, it was agreed that the title was too cumbersome and was therefore renamed the American Rheumatism Association (ARA). It is commonly assumed that the first scientific meeting of the ARA was held in Cleveland in 1934. On its program, however, the Cleveland meeting is listed as The First Annual Meeting of The American Association for the Study and Control of Rheumatic Diseases with Ernest E. Irons, President [4]! This situation continued annually until 1938 when, for the first time, the meeting is actually listed on the program as the meeting of the American Rheumatism Association. That meeting was held in San Francisco with William J. Kerr of San Francisco, President.‡ By 1938, meetings were a full day. Despite the original intent to keep the size of the association limited, membership had grown to 260. Scientific programs featured a striking variety

---

* Members of the ACCR: Llewellys F. Barker, Baltimore; Charles G. Bass, New Orleans; Russell L. Cecil, New York; A. Almon Fletcher, Toronto, Canada; Russell L. Haden, Kansas City; Philip S. Hench, Rochester, Minnesota, Secretary; Melvin S. Henderson, Rochester, Minnesota; Joseph L. Miller, Chicago; George A. Minot, Boston; Archer O'Reilly, St. Louis; Robert B. Osgood, Boston; Ralph Pemberton, Philadelphia, Chairman; Rea A. Smith, Los Agneles; Hans Zinsser, Boston.

† This meeting was held the day before the annual AMA Convention, as were all future scientific meetings until the early 1960s [10].

‡ The succession of the American Committee and of associations and their presidents are shown in Figure 1.2.

**PROGRAM**

# Conference on Rheumatic Diseases

AN OPEN MEETING SPONSORED BY

## The American Committee for the Control of Rheumatism

MONDAY, MAY 9, 1932, NINE O'CLOCK A.M. TO TWELVE NOON

Hotel Roosevelt, Room A, New Orleans

---

It is requested that papers be presented in abstract, not read. Time limit for papers will be 12 minutes. (For total discussion of any one paper time limit 8 minutes). Discussions of any paper by members of the audience are cordially invited.

---

1. Chairman's Introduction—Dr. Ralph Pemberton, Philadelphia

2. "Clinical and Economic Factors of Arthritis in 450 Ex-members of the Military Service."........ ...........................Dr. Philip B. Matz, Washington, D. C.

   Discussion: Dr. Wallace S. Duncan, Cleveland, Ohio, and Dr. Francis C. Hall, Boston.

3. "Relation of the Digestive Tract to Chronic Arthritis" ...........Dr. T. Preston White, Charlotte, North Carolina

4. "Gallbladder Disease in Chronic Infectious Arthritis: Results of Cholecystectomy"..............Dr. E. Starr Judd (and Dr. Philip S. Hench), Rochester, Minnesota

   Discussion (papers No. 3 and No. 4): Dr. R. Garfield Snyder, New York City, and Dr. A. R. Shands, Jr., Durham, North Carolina.

(a)

FIGURE 1.1.

of papers that involved possible etiologic factors, differential diagnosis, and medical and orthopedic treatment.

It is noteworthy that as early as 1926, Philip S. Hench of Mayo Clinic, following a year of observations in Germany, was the first appointed chief of an American academic division of arthritis to which residents and fellows were assigned [3]. Between 1929 and 1937, units for research and education were started by Walter Bauer at Harvard

5. "Climate Therapy for Chronic Arthritis: Results in 500 Cases"..............Dr. W. Paul Holbrook, Tucson, Arizona

6. "The Desensitization Treatment of Chronic Arthritis"...........Dr. James Craig Small, Philadelphia

7. "Intravenous Streptococcic Vaccine Therapy in Chronic Arthritis"...........Dr. Macnider Wetherby, Minneapolis

   Discussion (papers No. 5, No. 6 and No. 7): Dr. John W. Gray, Newark, New Jersey; Dr. Wm. J. Kerr, San Francisco, California, and Dr. O. O. Ashworth, Richmond, Virginia

   *Papers to be read if time permits*

8. "Sinus Infections as Silent Foci in Arthritis".........
   ................................Dr. R. Garfield Snyder, New York

9. "Degenerative Arthritis in Ilio-femoral Ligaments"..........................Dr. Edward K. Cravener, Boston

10. "The Joints in Infection".........Dr. Chester S. Keefer, and Dr. Walter K. Meyers, Boston ......................... .... .. .. ......

11. "The Arthritis Problem".........Dr. Millard Smith, Boston

12. "Classification of Osteo-arthritis"..............................
    ...........................Dr. Walter Gay Lough, New York City

---

You are cordially invited to visit the exhibit of the American Committee for The Control of Rheumatism to be held in Booths 1004, 1006, 1008 and 1010 in the Exhibit Hall.

Ralph Pemberton, M. D., Philadelphia, *Chairman*
Charles C. Bass, M. D., New Orleans
Russell L. Cecil, M. D., New York
A. Almon Fletcher, M. D., Toronto
Russell L. Haden, M. D., Cleveland
Melvin S. Henderson, M. D., Rochester, Minnesota

Joseph L. Miller, M. D., Chicago
George R. Minot, M. D., Boston
J. Archer O'Reilly, M. D., St. Louis
Robert B. Osgood, M. D., Boston
Cyrus C. Sturgis, M. D., Ann Arbor
Hans Zinsser, M. D., Boston
Philip S. Hench, M. D., Rochester, Minnesota, *Secretary*

(b)

**FIGURE 1.1.** *(Continued).*

University, Ralph H. Boots at Columbia University, Currier McEwen at New York University, and Richard Freyberg at the University of Michigan.

An early publication sponsored by the ACCR was *The Primer on Rheumatism, Chronic Arthritis* [11]. Published in *JAMA* in 1934, The Primer was aimed to help the practicing physicians in diagnosis and treatment of arthritis; its Editor was Edward Jordan, Associate Editor of *JAMA*. The second early publication was the

American Committee for Control of Rheumatism 1928-1934
Scientific Meetings 1932-1934
Ralph Pemberton, Chairman

American Association for the Study and Control of Rheumatic Diseases 1934-1937

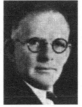 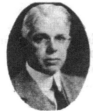 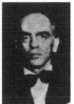

| Emest F. Irons | Russell L. Haden | Russell L. Cecil |
| 1934–35 | 1935–36 | 1936–37 |

American Rheumatism Association 1937-1960

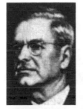 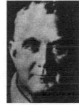 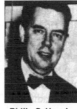 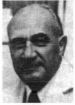 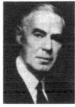

| William J. Kerr | Ralph Pemberton | Philip S. Hench | Ralph H. Boots | Loring T. Swain |
| 1937–38 | 1938–39 | 1939–40 | 1940–41 | 1941–42 |

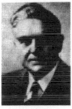 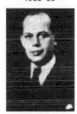 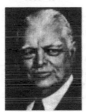 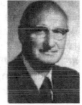 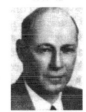

| W. Paul Holbrook | Walter Bauer | Robert M. Stecher | Richard H. Freyberg | T. Duckett Jones |
| 1942–45 | 1946–47 | 1947–48 | 1948–49 | 1949–50 |

    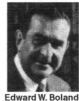

| Otto Steinbroker | Charles H. Slocumb | Currier McEwen | Charles Ragan | Edward W. Boland |
| 1950–51 | 1951–52 | 1952–53 | 1953–54 | 1954–55 |

| Charles L. Short | William D. Robinson | L. Maxwell Lockie | Joseph J. Bunim | Charley J. Smyth |
| 1955–56 | 1956–57 | 1957–58 | 1958–59 | 1959–60 |

**FIGURE 1.2.**

*Rheumatism Review* [12]. Directed to the clinical rheumatologist and investigator, it would provide reviews and updates of the English literature at 1-or 2-year intervals. First published in 1935 in the *Annals of Internal Medicine*, its editor was Dr. Hench.

Dr. Hench was well remembered for the classic, never-forgotten title of a paper he read at the 1940 ARA meeting: "An Oft-Recurring Disease of Joints (arthritis, peri-arthritis, para-arthritis) Apparently Producing No Articular Residues: Its Relationship to Angio-neural Arthrosis, Allergic Arthritis and Atrophic Arthritis. Report of 34 cases [3]. Some time later, Dr. Hench gave this recurring disease a new title, Palindromic Rheumatism, which was not a bad compromise [13].

There was no meeting of ARA during WW II. However, many leaders of the ARA were busily engaged in Army or Navy Centers for Arthritis or Rheumatic Fever, whereas another served as Consultant to the Surgeon General [14]. And then there was Currier McEwen, who was the Chief Consultant in Medicine for the entire European Theatre of Operations, and he had previously cooperated with Albert Einstein in creating positions at New York University and thus rescued some 20 Jewish physicians from the Nazis [15].

With the first reunion of the ARA in 1944, there was serious discussion of the need for financial support if the goals of ARA were to be met. After a national survey and consultation with the National Research Council, it was agreed that a new agency should be responsible for fundraising and disbursement of those funds for research and education, and that the ARA would continue as a separate medium for professional discussion of research and of advances in diagnosis and patient management. Thus, in 1948 the Arthritis and Rheumatism Foundation (A&RF) was formally established with W. Paul Holbrook of Tucson as President, and a well-known and respected business man Floyd B. Odlum as Chairman of the Board. Prominent members of the ARA constituted the Medical and Scientific Committee of A&RF's Board [3]. Seventeen years later, in 1965, "further unification" ensued when ARA, while preserving its functional independence, became a "Section" of the newly named Arthritis Foundation (see Figure 1.4).

A&RF's Research Fellowship Program and educational publications demonstrated early fulfillment of its objectives. A&RF's less obvious contribution was the availability of its administrative personnel to ARA. An outstanding example is one whose loyalty and untiring efforts extended from 1956 through 2007, Lynn Bonfiglio [10].

In 1949, an international congress hosted by the ARA and financially supported by A&RF was held in New York City. The meeting was a huge success. It commemorated two major events. First, it celebrated the inauguration of the enlarged International League Against Rheumatism (ILAR) [3]. In recent years, rheumatism societies of 13 European countries had organized La Ligue Internationale Contre le Rheumatisme. In 1944, rheumatism societies of nine North and South American countries, including the ARA, joined to create the Pan American League Against Rheumatism (PANLAR). At the New York meeting, PANLAR augmented ILAR to create an international league of two continents, the European and American. (In 1963, the rheumatism societies of Southeast Asia and Pacific Area [SEAPAL] became the third continental league of ILAR.)

The second major event of the New York meeting was the scientific program of papers read by worldwide experts. For the more than 500 international attendees, the real excitement occurred when Dr. Hench showed the movie of his rheumatoid arthritis patient failing an attempt to rise from a chair, and then easily rising from the chair 24 hours after the injection of cortisone [10]. The result was startling. A standing ovation followed. Respected American physicians, including Walter Bauer, came to the stage and extolled Dr. Hench's remarkable demonstration. What Dr. Bauer did not confess was that he had been given, for experimental use months earlier, adreno-corticotropic hormone. Because of his caution and conservatism, he failed to try it. It was still in his refrigerator, untouched!

Within a year after the New York meeting and with the help of intensive lobbying and testimony by Drs. Holbrook, President of A&RF, and Robert M. Stecher, President of ARA, the Omnibus Medical Research Act of 1950 was signed into law by President Truman. This act authorized the establishment of the National Institute of Arthritis and Metabolic Diseases (NIAMD) [3]. Although the A&RF and NIAMD would provide funds for research, the ARA would remain the major platform for discussion and for dissemination of information to the medical profession (Figure 1.3). It was also suggested that increasing philanthropic activity in the field of rheumatic diseases would be indispensable [16].

With the increasing abundance of information, it is not surprising that the ARA grew remarkably in size and importance. Two-day meetings supplemented later with interim sessions were required to offer adequate time for excellent papers.

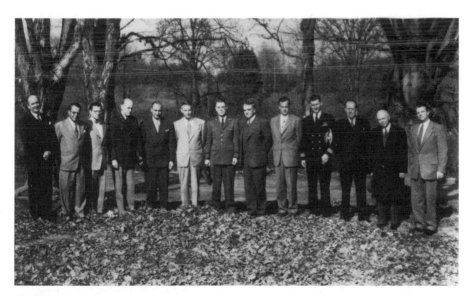

**FIGURE 1.3.** *First Meeting of the National Advisory Arthritis and Metabolic Diseases Council, November 15, 1950, Dr. William H. Sebrell, Jr., Dr. John A. Reed, Dr. Maxwell Wintrobe, Col. Paul S. Fancher, Dr. Richard H. Freyberg, Dr. Cecil J. Watson, Lt. Co. William D. Preston, Dr. W. Paul Holbrook, Dr. Alfred H. Lawton, Cmdr. J.S. Cowan, Mr. Wrston Howland, Mr. Clyde E. Wildman, and Dr. Floyd S. Draft.*

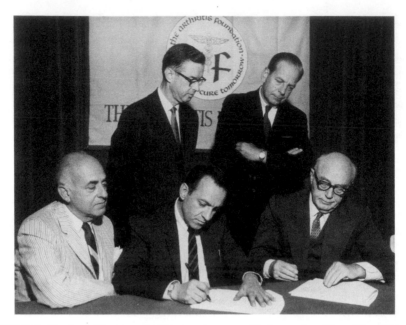

**FIGURE 1.4.** *Signing of the so-called Merger Agreement between the AF and the ARA, 1965. Standing: Howard F. Polley, William S. Clark, Sitting: Ephraim P. Engleman, Morris Ziff, Floyd B. Odlum.*

Membership in the 1950s had grown to about 1200. The attendees at meetings, however, were occasionally as few as 20–25% of the total membership [17]. And even though this caused concern, the small number in the audience encouraged lively discussion. In private rooms where the Executive Committees met, discussions were lively, and they could be acrimonious. An example of that occurred at the San Francisco meeting of 1954 [10].

Joseph L. Hollander of Philadelphia had just given a thorough report of his Committee on the Desirability and Feasibility of an American Journal on Arthritis and Rheumatism. After careful study of the pros and cons, his Committee's unanimous recommendation was that the journal is both desirable and feasible. In no uncertain terms, the Executive Committee's members, including some past presidents, objected vociferously. There was already too much competition, "and anyway, there was too little editorial talent in the ARA." Dr. Hollander was asked to evaluate these and other criticisms, but instead he resigned his Chairmanship, convinced that a fresh approach was indicated. And so, soon thereafter, Dr. Freyberg was appointed as Chair. It was 4 years later when the Journal was finally approved. In 1958, the first issue of *Arthritis and Rheumatism* was published with William S. Clark as its Editor [18].

Not all that took place at annual meetings was necessarily serious business. Related events often provided light-hearted entertainment. For example, and again in San Francisco, a ferryboat excursion provided not only a sightseeing cruise of the San Francisco Bay but also dinner and drinks [10]. The walls of the boat were filled with signs extolling Walter Bauer's favorite drug. Instead of Bayer's Aspirin, the signs read Bauer's Aspirin. A certain distinguished ARA member had a few too many drinks and had to be carried off the boat. At 8 a.m. the following morning, he was the first speaker at the Session on Clinical Research. Holding tightly on the podium, his opening comment was, "I still feel the rocking of that boat! I seem to have a heavy head." The title of his paper was "Gold Therapy in Rheumatoid Arthritis."

By 1970, the purposes of the pioneers of rheumatology were not only met but even exceeded. A revised Nomenclature and Classification had been approved [19]. Diagnostic criteria for rheumatoid arthritis had been proposed [20,21]. The early publication, *The Primer*, was enlarged from 8 to 71 pages and on its way to more [3]. The highly regarded educational publication, *The Rheumatism Review*, would fulfill its purpose with its 25th and final edition. Excellent material increased the issues of the journal *Arthritis and Rheumatism* from 6 to 12 per year. The first collection of lantern slides for teaching purposes had been offered to physicians. ARA membership continued its growth from 100 to 2300. Interest developed for collaboration with allied health professionals. Last, but surely not least, and for the first time, a woman was elected to the presidency of ARA: Marian W. Ropes of Boston [10].

## REFERENCES

1. Billings F. Chronic focal infections and their etiologic relation to arthritis and nephritis. Arch Intern Med 1912;9:484–498.
2. Dawson MH, Boots RH. Recent studies in rheumatoid (chronic infectious, atrophic) arthritis. N Engl J Med 1933;208:1030–1035.
3. Smyth CJ, Freyberg RH, McEwen C. History of Rheumatology in the United States. Alpharetta, GA: Arthritis Foundation; 1985.
4. Stecher RM. American Rheumatism Association: Its origins, development and maturity. Arthritis Rheum 1958;1:4–19.
5. Pemberton R, Foster GL. Studies on arthritis in the army, based on 400 cases. Arch Intern Med 1920;25:243.
6. Pemberton R. The control of rheumatism (editorial). JAMA 1928;91:30–31.
7. Nichols EH, Richardson FL. Arthritis deformans. J Med Res 1909;21:149–205.
8. Hench PS, et al. Rheumatism and arthritis: Review of American and English literature for 1940 (Eighth Rheumatism Review). Ann Intern Med 1941;15:1002.
9. A conference on rheumatic diseases. JAMA 1932;99:1020–1022.
10. Engleman EP. Personal observation.
11. American Medical Association. Primer on rheumatism. Chicago, IL: American Medical Association; 1934.
12. Hench, PS, Bauer W, Fletcher AA, et al. The present status of the problem of rheumatism: A review of recent American and English literature on "rheumatism" and arthritis. Ann Intern Med 1935;8:1315–1374, 1495–1555, 1556–1580.
13. Hench PS, Rosenberg EF. Palindromic rheumatism. Arch Intern Med 1944;73:293–321.
14. Hench PS, Boland EW. The management of chronic arthritis and other rheumatic diseases among soldiers of the United States Army. Ann Intern Med 1946;24:808–825.

15. Block MM, Block SR. In memoriam. Currier McEwen, MD. Arthritis Rheum 2003; 48:2739–2740.

16. Engleman EP. The crusade against arthritis: The role of the American Rheumatism Association. Arthritis Rheum 1963;6:311–316.

17. Engleman EP. President's message. Arthritis Rheum 1963;5:668–669.

18. Clark WS. Arthritis and rheumatism: Official journal of the American Rheumatism Association (editorial). Arthritis Rheum 1958;1:1–3.

19. Blumberg B, Bunim JJ, Calkins E, et al. ARA nomenclature and classification of arthritis and rheumatism (tentative). Arthritis Rheum 1964;7:93–97.

20. Ropes MW, Bennett GA, Cobb S, et al. Proposed diagnostic criteria for rheumatoid arthritis. Bull Rheum Dis 1956;7:121–124.

21. Ropes, MW, Bennett GA, Cobb S, et al. Revision of diagnostic criteria for rheumatoid arthritis. Bull Rheum Dis 1958;9:175–176.

# Chapter 2

# History of the ACR: After 1970

**Charles L. Christian**

*University of Florida School of Medicine, Gainesville, FL*

This chapter will weigh factors that have changed the American College of Rheumatology (ACR) over the past 38 years, but because some of these factors began to evolve earlier, it is appropriate to return (briefly) to the beginning and consider who the early members of the ACR were. They were captured in a photograph dated June 1937 (Figure 2.1). The occasion was an annual meeting of the Society in Atlantic City; this was the year that the name "American Rheumatism Asssociation" (ARA) was officially adopted. A year later, when the organization met in San Francisco, was the first time that the new name appeared on the program. (The photographer mistakenly labeled the group as the "National American Rheumatic Association.")

The early members shared several characteristics: First, the small number (75) relative to current ACR membership (7012). Second, most were internists; some of them became interested in arthritis because a family member or friend was affected and they realized that for many patients the course of disease was inexorable, the emphasis in names of Committees antecedent to ARA was "control" of arthritis. In the photo, the earliest leaders of the ARA are clustered in the front row; scattered throughout are a total of 11 who served as presidents of the Society. Maybe a few of them were beginning to limit their practice to patients with rheumatic disease, but most considered themselves general internists. There was one orthopedic surgeon (Robert Osgood), a couple of pathologists, and a pediatrician. Third, most of the early

*The ACR at 75: A Diamond Jubilee*
Copyright © 2009 by John Wiley & Sons, Inc.

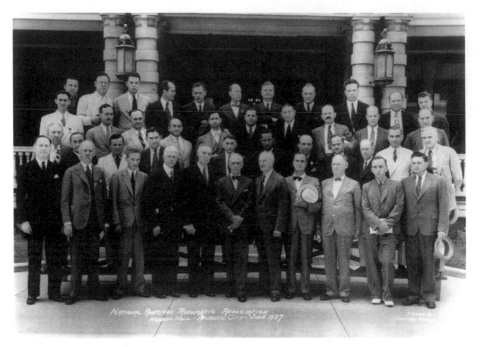

**FIGURE 2.1.** *Photograph of Attendees at Meeting of the "National American Rheumatic (sic) Association. Atlantic City, New Jersey 1937.*

> **Front row**: 1& 2 (?)*, 3 A.A. Fletcher, 4 Ernest Irons, 5 Loring Swain, 6 Russell Cecil, 7 Homer Swift, 8, Ralph Pemberton, 9 (?). 10 Lemoyne Kelly, 11 W. Paul Holbrook
>
> **Second row**: 12 (?), 13 Otto Steinbrocker, 14,–16 (?), 17 J.G. Kuhns, 18 T.P. White, 19 unknown, 20 James Rinehart, 21 L. Speare, 22 John Gray,
>
> **Third row**: 23 (?), 24 William Ishmael, 25 Murray Angevine, 26 Taylor, 27 L.Maxwell Lockie, 28–31 (?), 32 Charles Short, 33 (?)
>
> **Back Row**: 34–35 (?), 36 Phillip Hench, 37 Walter Bauer, 38 unknown, 39 Robert Osgood, 40 M. Henry Dawson, 41 Ralph Boots, 42–43 (?), 44 Connie Traeger * (?) name unknown

members lived in the northeast. Fourth, there were no women, and last, there were only two people who could be identified as laboratory scientists: Homer Swift in the front row and M. Henry Dawson near the middle of the back row. Both men had connections to the Rockefeller Institute. Swift spent his entire professional life there studying the role of streptococci in rheumatic fever (ARA presidents Ralph Boots and Currier McEwen had been trainees in his laboratory). Dawson, who was an associate of Oswald T. Avery, was involved in early studies of the pneumococcal transforming factor; he came to Columbia; in 1929 as Director of the Faulkner Arthritis Clinic. There was a diaspora of talent, in addition to those already noted, from Rockefeller Institute to other New York institutions; Alphonse R. Dochez and Michael Heidelberger to Columbia; and William S. Tillett to New York University (NYU) (Chair of Medicine). In a sense, this was analogous to the more recent scattering of Henry Kunkel's scientific progeny to rheumatology programs here and abroad.

**TABLE 2.1    ACR (ARA) Membership**

| Year | 1934 | 1944 | 1954 | 1964 | 1974 | 1984 | 1994 | 2004 | 2008 |
|---|---|---|---|---|---|---|---|---|---|
| Members | 75 | 280 | 908 | 1615 | 2262 | 4200 | 5350 | 6825 | 7012 |

Three people in the photo were participants in the earliest example of interinstitutional rheumatic disease research; this involved Boots and Dawson at Columbia and Cecil at Cornell. Cecil and his bacteriology colleagues (Nicholls and Stainsby at Bellevue) were reporting isolation of beta hemolytic streptococci from blood and joints of rheumatoid patients and host humoral immunity to the bacteria; this finding seemed to support the "foci of infection" hypothesis (referred to earlier) and the use of a popular alternative term for rheumatoid arthritis, "chronic infectious arthritis" [1,2]. Because Boots and Dawson could not confirm the bacterial isolations [3], a blinded collaboration was organized. Blood specimens from 25 rheumatoid patients and 25 controls were sent from Columbia to Cecil. The studies' conclusions were as follows: 1) The isolation of bacteria was the result of intralaboratory contamination, but 2) streptococcal agglutination was real, 80% of rheumatoid patients (but no controls) were positive [4]. The latter was indication of a substance in sera that would later be called "rheumatoid factor."

Now, focusing on changes in the ACR after 1970, membership at decade intervals is summarized in Table 2.1. Membership has increased almost 100-fold from the beginning, and, since 1970, 4-fold. Attendance at annual ACR meetings (5-year intervals from 1980) are summarized in Table 2.2. Recording of international attendance did not begin until 1993; for a few years, it did not exceed 30% but, since 1995, it has been in the 50–60% range. The internationalization of medicine and science is one of the forces that has contributed to the growth of the ACR (Table 2.3).

Going back in time, in 1948 there was a "burst" of new information regarding the role of the immune systems in the pathogenesis of rheumatic disease; this attracted to the field a large cadre of investigators who, over the past half-century, have enormously enlarged our knowledge of subjects such as immunogenetics, immune regulation, autoimmunity, and immune complex disease. The dramatic effect of cortisone treatment of patients with rheumatoid arthritis in 1949 likewise enhanced scientific inquiry relative to the field, and it gave a boost to passage of the Omnibus Medical Research Act of 1950, which enabled large-scale expansion of programs of the National Institutes of Health (NIH). Dr. Engleman has summarized the role of ACR leadership in formation of the Arthritis and Rheumatism Foundation (A&RF). The Foundation played a broad advocacy role in the interest of patients, but its primary mission from its beginning, which overlaps interests of ACR, was to support research manpower training. The Fellowship Program was launched in 1951 with an allocation of $33,500 for support of seven trainees; at the 25-year mark of its history, more than

**TABLE 2.2    Attendance at ACR & ARHP Annual Meetings**

| Year | 1980 | 1985 | 1990 | 1995 | 2000 | 2005 | 2008 |
|---|---|---|---|---|---|---|---|
| ACR | 1676 | 1932 | 2839 | 4423 | 7302 | 8226 | 10092 |
| ARHP | 342 | 392 | 535 | 602 | 614 | 616 | 933 |

**TABLE 2.3  "Growth Factors" for ACR**

Developments 1928 to 1948
  Recognition of Rheumatism as a category of disease
  Development of Nomenclature and Classification
  Early Publications: Primer, Rheumatism Reviews
Developments 1948-1950
  Arthritis & Rheumatism Foundation established (1949)
  Corticosteroid Therapy for Rheumatoid Arthritis
  Omnibus Medical Research Act  (US Congress)
    National Institute of Arthritis and Metabolic Diseases
    NIH Clinical Center in Bethesda
    Expanded Funding of Extra-mural Research Support
Developments After 1950
  Arthritis & Rheumatism (Journal) initiated (1958)
  New Insights Re; immunopathogenesis of Rheumatic Diseases
  ABIM Approval of Rheumatology Board Certification (1971)
  Approval of Arthritis Act US Congress (1975)
    Multi-Purpose Arthritis Centers
    Research Epidemiology Programs
    Support of Data Systems Development
  New Therapies, Including Prosthetic Arthoplasties
  Global Character of Medicine and Biomedical Research
  ARA Organized as a Separate Professional Society  (1985)
  Development of Research & Education Fund

$9 million had funded training of 371 fellows, 31 of that group were directors of major rheumatic disease programs.

Developments after 1950 that had bearing on the growth of the ACR include the following: 1) the foundation of *Arthritis & Rheumatism* (A&R) (ACR's official journal) in 1958,; 2) approval of Board Certification in Rheumatology by the American Board of Internal Medicine (ABIM) (1971), first exam 1972 [both *A&R* and Board Certification were favorite projects of Joseph Lee Hollander, ARA President 1961–1962. From personal experience, the writer knows that he essentially hand-picked the first 3 Editors of *A&R*.], 3) the Arthritis Act (1975) authorized increased NIH support of epidemiology and data systems research and enabled establishment of multipurpose arthritis centers, and 4) new insights regarding molecular bases for rheumatic disease and new therapeutic strategies have clearly expanded the scope and mission of rheumatology.

The reconfiguration of the ACR and the development of ACR as an independent professional society is probably the most potent of growth factors. Figure 2.2 summarizes schematically the changing inter-relationships of the ACR, Arthritis Foundation, Association of Rheumatology Health Professionals (ARHP), and their organizational antecedents.

Dr. Engleman has reviewed the roles that ARA members played in the creation of the Arthritis & Rheumatism Foundation: The CEO of the Foundation (Floyd B. Odium) was a patient of Richard Freyberg's; he served in that role for almost four decades. The chief administrator of the Foundation was General George C. Kenny,

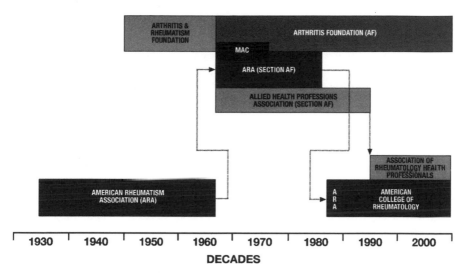

**FIGURE 2.2.** *Schematic Representation of Administrative Interactions Between: ACR, AHRP & AF and Their Antecedent Organizations.*

who was General Macarthur's Commander of Allied Air Forces in the Southwest Pacific Area 1942–1945. The governing body of the Foundation was a group of nine regional delegates. The borders of the nine regions were thought to be based on the geographic distribution of U.S. Army supply commands; to some leaders of the ARA, the delegates seemed to be more fixed on inter-regional disputes than on running a foundation. In 1964–1966, during the presidencies of Howard F. Polley and Morris Ziff, the ARA and A&RF were reorganized, the A&RF became the Arthritis Foundation, Dr. William S. Clark was elected its President and the ARA, while maintaining functional independence, became a "Section" of the Foundation. A Medical Advisory Committee (MAC) composed of both Arthritis Foundation (AF) and American Rheumatism Association (ARA) leadership duplicated some of the functions of the two organizations. After a decade (in 1976), it was eliminated and the two parts were more formally merged at which time Clifford Clark became President and CEO of the Foundation.

Two decades after the merged relationship of the two organizations, some problems were beginning to surface. First, ACR membership had doubled, reflecting the growth of rheumatology as a clinical discipline; these members were not wholly satisfied with the degree of practice-related issues being pursued. There was risk that the more clinically oriented members might organize their own society. Second, the Arthritis Foundation was expressing concern that pursuit of practice-related programs might jeopardize its 501(c)3 tax status. Third, there were financial issues; the ARA programs generated increasing sums, but its leaders were frustrated by the Foundation's accounting procedures. San Francisco was the host of the International Congress on Rheumatic Diseases in 1977. The Finance Committee for the Congress was successful in generating a record sum of money, with the expectations that any income over cost would be applied to educational endeavors. This was a "bone of contention." Last, there were also issues of style and personality; Clifford Clark and his deputy (Vance Lockhart) brought important management skills to the Foundation, but they never quite understood the ARA. They were sometimes frustrated by what "the doctors" wanted to do. The final and deciding event was an ultimatum from Clifford Clark to Eng Tan (ARA President 1984–1985) to cease all activities that might alter the Foundation's tax status. At the time of its annual meeting in 1985, the ARA voted to proceed with plans to organize as a free-standing professional society. William Kelley who was then Secretary conducted negotiations for separation with great distinction and later, during his presidency (1986–1987), was instrumental in recruiting Mark Andrejeski as ARA Executive Vice President. Two years later (1988), the ARA membership supported the change of name to ACR, and in 1994, the Allied Health Professions Association, which had remained as a Section of the Arthritis Foundation, voted to join the ACR and change its name to the Association of Rheumatology Health Professionals.

The case has been made that the independence of the ACR was a powerful growth factor, but the Arthritis Foundation has also prospered; the two organizations are functionally not different than they were before the separation. They share missions, purpose, and advocacy for all patients with rheumatic disease. Together (including the ACR's Research & Education Foundation), they are the force for generation of public support of rheumatic disease research and training.

Finally, a comment about someone who was never an officer of ARA/ACR but who played some interesting and vital roles in affairs of the organization and its inter-relationships with other entities. William S. Clark trained with Dr. Walter Bauer (ARA President, 1946–1947), and he remained at the Massachusetts General Hospital for several years before joining the faculty of Case Western Reserve University College of Medicine. At the time of the Ninth International Congress on Rheumatic Diseases in Toronto (1957), it was known that Bill Clark would be the first Editor of *Arthritis & Rheumatism*, which was to be launched a year later. During this interval, Basil O'Connor (President of the March of Dimes Foundation), who was aware that poliomyelitis was being removed from the list of unsolved medical problems in America, had a conversation with Floyd Odlum, and the two of them agreed to have arthritis added to the mission of the March of Dimes. Bill Clark was invited to serve as the Medical Director for rheumatic disease programs of the March of Dimes.

Not all the leadership personnel of the ARA liked this arrangement. When the Society met next in San Francisco, June 1958, Bill Clark got some fairly rough treatment. A preeminent founder of ARA accused him of being a traitor; nevertheless, for approximately 5 years, under Bill Clark's directorship, the March of Dimes supported arthritis research and treatment programs. Two of his initiatives stand out as follows: 1) the development of multidisciplinary arthritis centers and 2) recognition and support of the allied health professions, which were antecedent to foundation of AHRP. These two programs were continued by the Arthritis Foundation with interim support from the March of Dimes. Ephraim Engleman remembers being in an informal meeting with Floyd Odlum and Basil O'Connor in a room at the Mark Hopkins Hotel where procedural and financial details were agreed upon. Figure 2.3 is

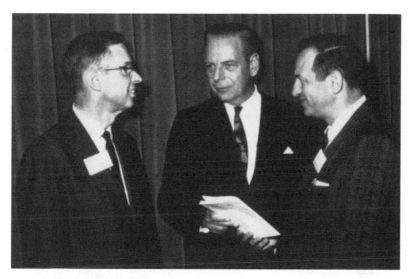

**FIGURE 2.3.** *Photograph, Including From Left to Right: Howard F. Polley (ARA President 1964–65), William S. Clark (President Arthritis Foundation) and Morris Ziff (ARA President 1965–66), Taken 1965 at time of Re-Organization of the Arthritis Foundation and Inclusion of ACR as a Section of the Foundation.*

a photograph of William Clark with presidents Morris Ziff and Howard Polley, which signified the role ARA leaders played in the reorganization of the Foundation and the selection of Bill Clark as its President.

Bill Clark was a mentor of this writer and others, who include Mart Mannik; this leads to the final anecdote to illustrate the power of unintended consequences. Mart was a medical student about the same time that Bill Clark arrived at Case Western Reserve. All students were required to identify a faculty member who could guide them in a research experience over the ensuing 4 years. Mart thought metabolic bone disease was interesting but could not identify a sponsor relative to that, then he considered a project in hematology, but the faculty leader in that area already had a few students signed up. Finally Mart's assigned faculty advisor told him that there was new person (Bill Clark) on the faculty, he had no idea what his specialty interests were, but because he was so recently arrived, he might be uncommitted as a faculty sponsor. A couple of years later, I met Mart when, as a student, he was presenting a paper at an Interim Meeting of the ARA.

In conclusion, multiple developments have contributed to the growth and success of the ACR. Two other factors—not yet mentioned—have been critically important as follows: 1) the wisdom and energy of a succession of elected officers who have given much more of their time and effort to the organization than did their predecessors a generation ago and 2) the enlightened leadership of Mark Andrejeski (Executive Vice President) over the past two decades. The odyssey of the ACR over 75 years is short of its destination, but many interesting things have happened, and there is more to come.

## REFERENCES

1. Cecil RL, Nicholls EE, Stainsby WJ. The bacteriology of the blood and joints in chronic infections arthritis. Arch Intern Med 1929;43:571–605.
2. Cecil RL, Nicholls EE, Stainsby WJ. The etiology of rheumatoid arthritis. Am J Med Sci 1931;181:12–25.
3. Dawson MH, Olmstead M, Boots RH. Bacteriologic investigations of blood, synovial fluid and subcutaneous nodules in rheumatoid (chronic infectious) arthritis. Arch Intern Med 1932;49:173–180.
4. Dawson MH, Olmstead M, Boots RH. Agglutination reactions in rheumatoid arthritis. II. The nature and significance of agglutination reactions with streptococcal hemolyticus. J Immunol 1932;23:205–228.

# Chapter 3

# The History of the Association of Rheumatology Health Professionals (ARHP)*

**Teresa J. Brady**

*Center for Disease Control, Arthritis Program, Atlanta, GA*

## 3.1 INTRODUCTION

The Association of Rheumatology Health Professionals (ARHP) is a professional association of a wide array of health professionals involved in rheumatology research, education, and care. From its early roots as the Paramedical Section of the Medical Council of the Arthritis Foundation to its current position as a division within the American College of Rheumatology (ACR), the ARHP has remained true to its essential values of multidisciplinary/interdisciplinary collaborations, and improving the lives of people with arthritis. Through its multitude of name changes and organizational homes (the Arthritis Foundation 1965–1993, ACR 1994

---

*This findings and conclusions in this article are those of the author and do not necessarily represent the views of the Centers for Disease Control and Prevention.

---

**TABLE 3.1. Organizational Mission**

1967: Purposes of the "Paramedical Section of the Medical Council of the Arthritis Foundation": (extracted from inaugural Rules of Procedure, ratified 1967) [1]:

1) establishment of interdisciplinary communication about comprehensive services, teaching, and research in the rheumatic and connective tissue diseases;

2) stimulation and promotion of ideas and activities within and among the respective disciplines in relation to these diseases;

3) promotion of public understanding of the comprehensive approaches to the care of persons with these diseases.

2009: Purposes of the Association of Rheumatology Health Professionals: (Extracted from Rules of Procedure approved 2007) [2]:
Using programs of education, practice, research, and advocacy, the Association of Rheumatology Health Professionals will advance the knowledge and skills of health professionals in the area of rheumatology and will improve their understanding and management of the physical, emotional, psychological, and cultural factors influencing health in order to improve the health outcomes for people with or at risk for rheumatic disease and musculoskeletal conditions.

to present), the core strengths of the organization remain constant. As demonstrated in Table 3.1, the charter members' vision emphasized interdisciplinary communication and cross-fertilization of ideas in comprehensive approaches to rheumatology care, teaching, and research. These foci remain critical today (Table 3.1).

Rather than present a chronological history of the organization, this chapter will review sentinel accomplishments and events that highlight key strengths of the organization since its inception. Highlights include producing multiple educational products and practice tools, convening a scientific meeting each year, establishing the journal *Arthritis Care and Research* as the premier locus for rheumatology health professions and clinical care research, and merging with the American College of Rheumatology. Table 3.2 [2] includes a chronological history of selected events within ARHP and within the environment ARHP was functioning in.

## 3.2 EVOLUTION FROM PARAMEDICAL SECTION TO ASSOCIATION OF RHEUMATOLOGY HEALTH PROFESSIONALS

At first glance, the early frequent name changes may seem trivial; however, they reflect the organization's evolving identity and professionalism. Presidents leading the organization at the time of these name changes have identified them as significant achievements of their presidency [3,4]. The name Paramedical Section was assigned by the Arthritis Foundation Bylaws when the group was created, and it was unpopular with members from the beginning [5]. In 1968, shortly after the organization was established, members catalyzed a name change to the Allied

**TABLE 3.2. Timeline of Selected ARHP Milestones and Environmental Events**

| Organizational Milestones | | Environmental Events |
|---|---|---|
| Planning committee convened to establish "Paramedical Section." | 1965 | Medicare created. |
| First Membership and Annual Meeting held. | 1966 | |
| First Rules of Procedure ratified, formally establishing the "Paramedical Section" of the Medical Council of the Arthritis Foundation. | 1967 | |
| First President elected. | | |
| Membership and Education Committees established. | | |
| First issue of Newsletter published. | | |
| Name changed to Allied Health Professions (AHP) Section. | 1968 | |
| Research committee established. | | |
| Publications committee established. | 1969 | |
| | 1970 | First AHP representative to Arthritis Foundation (AF) Fellowship Committee. |
| | 1972 | First Rheumatology Subspecialty Board examination. |
| | 1973 | First AHP Fellowship awarded by AF. |
| | 1974 | Arthritis Act passed by congress (signed into law January 1975). |
| Self-Help Manual published. | 1975 | National Commission on Arthritis and Related Musculoskeletal Diseases created. |
| | 1976 | National Arthritis Advisory Board created. |
| | 1977 | NIH supported Multipurpose Arthritis Centers (MAC) funded. |
| Name changed to Arthritis Health Professions Section. | 1978 | Arthritis Foundation begins to fund AHP research grants. |
| Name changed to Arthritis Health Professions Association (AHPA) | 1980 | |
| Regional Meetings began. | | |
| Teaching Slide Collection produced | | |
| Containing Education Units (CEUs) available at Annual Scientific Meeting for first time. | 1981 | |
| Educational Materials Exhibit created. | | |
| ARA and AHPA Annual Scientific Meeting integrated. | 1982 | |
| Scholarship Award created. | | |

(continued)

**TABLE 3.2.** *(Continued)*

| Year | Organizational Milestones | Environmental Events |
|---|---|---|
| 1983 | Addie Thomas Service award created. Outcome Standards for Rheumatology Nursing published. First Physician President of AHPA. | American Rheumatism Association celebrates 50th Anniversary. |
| 1984 | Scholarship Award created. | |
| 1985 | Rheumatology Review Course/State of the Art Course initiated. Physical Therapy Standards published and adopted by AHPA. | National Institutes of Health establishes National Institute of Arthritis, Musculoskeletal, and Skin Diseases. |
| 1986 | Occupational Therapy Role and Function paper published. New Rules of Procedures (ROPs) approved; create Member Services and Practice Committee. | ARA separates from the Arthritis Foundation. Research and Education Foundation established. |
| 1987 | Home Study course created. Adapt-Ability: An Arthritis Fashion Show presented at annual meeting. | |
| 1988 | First issue of *Arthritis Care and Research* published. | ARA renamed American College of Rheumatology. AF and ACR sign memorandum of agreement. |
| 1989 | Model Core Curriculum produced. Cooking in Comfort for People with Arthritis show at annual meeting. | |
| 1994 | First special issue of *Arthritis Care & Research.* First international member elected. President of AHPA. Organization separates from the Arthritis Foundation, becomes the Association of Rheumatology Health Professionals, A Division of ACR. | |
| 1995 | Lifetime Achievement Award established. | |
| 1996 | Clinical Care in the Rheumatic Diseases published. | |
| 1999 | | Release of the National Arthritis Action Plan: A Public Health Strategy. First congressional appropriation for a public health approach for arthritis. |
| 2003 | Web-based case studies published on website. Clinical Master Award established. | ACR produces Position Statement on Multidisciplinary Care. |
| 2007 | Ann Kunkel Advocacy Award established. | |
| 2008 | Online NP/PA Postgraduate Rheumatology Training Program released. ROP changes are proposed to integrate select committees with ACR counterparts. | |

Health Professions Section to reflect the professional stature of the membership. Ten years later, to be inclusive of all professions, the name was changed to Arthritis Health Professions Section, and subsequently Arthritis Health Professions Association (AHPA) [5]. The organization retained the AHPA name until it joined the ACR in 1994 and became the Association of Rheumatology Health Professionals. To avoid confusion, the organization will be referred to as the ARHP for this brief history.

## 3.3  EDUCATIONAL PRODUCTS AND PRACTICE TOOLS

The organization, regardless of name, has a strong tradition of producing high-quality, clinically relevant educational materials and practice tools. Early educational materials, developed in the late 1960s, included a booklet on home care and a manual for professionals working with patients with arthritis; both documents were published and distributed by the Arthritis Foundation [5]. As the organization's sophistication grew, so did the sophistication of the educational products: including a self-help manual originally produced in 1974, a "how to" manual for patient education, a home study course (1987), the model core curriculum for teaching health professionals (1988), [1] and the web-based case studies developed in the early 2000s. Educational products are always matched to the needs of the membership. In the late 1970s, long before computers and Microsoft PowerPoint, members needed slides for teaching both patients and students. The teaching slide collection was therefore produced. More recently, as the role of nurse practitioners (NPs) and physician assistants (PAs) increased in rheumatology, the online rheumatology training program for NPs and PAs was developed. All these educational materials had the same overarching goal: to enable health professionals to provide high-quality education and care to people living with arthritis.

A signature educational product is the *Clinical Care in the Rheumatic Diseases*, which was first published in 1996. This text was produced as a companion to the *Primer on the Rheumatic Diseases*, and it was designed to collate, into a single publication, state-of-the-art techniques for the clinical care of people with arthritis. The third edition is currently in widespread use both nationally and internationally.

A key focus in the 1980s was role clarification among the professions and explaining the role of health professionals in rheumatology care. This effort lead to the development of the outcome standards for rheumatology nursing (1983) [6], competencies for physical therapists in rheumatology (1985) [7], and a paper outlining the role of and function of occupational therapists in rheumatology (1986) [8]. Most of these were coproduced with the corresponding discipline-specific professional organization. In the 1990s, briefing papers were prepared on the role of advanced practice nurses, occupational therapists, physical therapists, physician assistants, psychologists, registered nurses, rheumatologists, social workers, and the interdisciplinary team in the management of patients with rheumatic diseases [9]. In 2003, in collaboration with ACR, a position paper on multidisciplinary care was developed [10].

## 3.4    ANNUAL SCIENTIFIC MEETING

ARHP's signature event is the Annual Scientific Meeting, held in conjunction with the ACR Annual Scientific Meeting. Since the beginning, ARHP has emphasized bringing multidisciplinary health professionals together to exchange ideas through the presentation of scientific papers as well as the more informal, but equally stimulating "hallway conversations." The first annual meeting took place in 1966, before the organization was officially established [1]. In the 1980s, the program evolved from just being colocated with the ACR meeting to being increasingly integrated; currently, there is minimal distinction between ARHP- and ACR-sponsored sessions. Attendance at the Annual Scientific Meetings has grown from less than 100 professionals in the early days to over 1000 at the 43rd annual meeting in 2008 [11].

More noteworthy than the increasing attendance has been the increase in quality of the science presented. Although the meetings in the early days presented more of the art of clinical care, strong science, both experimental and applied, now predominates [12]. This increase in quality is a reflection of the increase in sophistication of researchers working in rheumatology, which is driven primarily by rheumatology health professional research funding available from the National Institutes of Health, the Arthritis Foundation [1,5], and, in recent years, the ACR's Research and Education Foundation.

## 3.5    ARTHRITIS CARE AND RESEARCH

Although the annual scientific meeting is an organizational highlight, the flagship product of ARHP is unquestionably *Arthritis Care & Research (AC&R)*, which is the division's professional journal. Discussions about the need for a journal to create a singular publication location for the increasingly high quality and quantity of research produced by rheumatology health professionals began in the late 1970s. Exploring the feasibility of producing a journal formally began in 1983, and the first issue was published in 1988. Part of the early uncertainty about producing a journal was financial; equally important was concern about whether a sufficient supply of high-quality research would be submitted. Originally, four issues were published each year. This number increased to six issues per year in 1996, and in 2009, the journal began monthly publication to meet the volume of high-quality research being submitted. The journal has become the leading source for cutting-edge rheumatology health professions and clinical care research.

The journal benefited from strong editorial leadership and organizational commitment. The early history was rocky because financial viability was uncertain, and stabilizing the journal financing was a predominant issue in the 1990s. However, with the move of the organization to ACR and the creation of *AC&R* as a section of *Arthritis & Rheumatism (A&R)*, the stellar original journal of the college, *Arthritis Care and Research* has a strong financial base and a bright future. The union with *A&R* has facilitated role clarification between the college's two journals and expansion of *AC&R*'s mission to increase coverage of broader clinical care issues, health economics, epidemiology, and public health research.

## 3.6 THE MERGER WITH ACR

As ACR celebrates its 75th anniversary and ARHP nears its 45th anniversary, it is important to reflect not only on the ARHP's pivotal accomplishments but also an event of singular importance, the merger of ARHP into ACR. ARHP was created at the time that the American Rheumatism Association (ARA), which was the precursor to ACR, and the Arthritis Foundation merged in 1965 [1]. ARHP remained within the Arthritis Foundation when ARA left to create an independent organization, the ACR, in 1986 [5]. Assessing both the merits of merging two professional associations and the challenges of merging a predominantly health professional organization with a predominately physician organization, ARHP chose to join ACR in 1994 [13]. This merger has strengthened both organizations, fostered increased interdisciplinary communication and care, and modeled strong physician–health professional partnerships in addressing the challenges of arthritis. In contrast to initial concerns, health professionals have remained active participants in the Arthritis Foundation while also establishing their valuable role on ACR committees. The merged organizations are both thriving and demonstrate broad interdisciplinary collaboration even in their routine operations.

## 3.7 CONCLUSION

ARHP has evolved from its status as a paraprofessional section of the Arthritis Foundation to a professional division of the ACR. Over time, individual members increased the sophistication of their research and clinical skills. The sophistication of the organization's educational products, annual scientific meetings, and publications increased in parallel. The merger with ACR has allowed ARHP to thrive while making considerable contribution to ACR.

It is noteworthy that, for most of the more than 1100 members, ARHP is their secondary professional association; many also belong to their discipline-specific professional association. Despite this situation, ARHP members have devoted many hours of volunteer labor to ARHP, over many years of active involvement. When past presidents were asked to reflect on what kept them motivated to invest time and energy into ARHP, several themes emerged. Consistent with the charter members' vision, the opportunity for collaboration across disciplines and a spirit of productivity that transcended personal or disciplinary agendas were key reasons that these organizational leaders remained committed over time. These leaders also identified opportunities for professional growth and mentoring, fine friendships with dedicated and insightful colleagues, and the opportunity to provide tangible benefits to people with arthritis as important motivators. ARHP provides a tantalizing mixture of professional development, interdisciplinary collaboration, and meaningful involvement that makes it unique in the professional lives of active members.

## REFERENCES

1. Riggs GK. Arthritis Health Professions Association. In: History of Rheumatology in the United States. (Smythe CJ, Freyberg RH, and McEwen C. Eds.). Atlanta, GA: Arthritis Foundation; 1985, pp. 95–103.
2. Association of Rheumatology Health Professionals. Rules of procedure. Revised August 17, 2007.
3. Berthold Wolfe B. Personal communication. February 2005.
4. Pigg Janice S. Personal communication, November 2008.
5. Partridge AJ, Riggs GK. The History of the Arthritis Health Professions Association 1965–1990. Atlanta, GA: Arthritis Foundation; 1990.
6. Arthritis Foundation. Outcome Standards for Rheumatology Nursing Practice. American Nursing Association, Division of Medical and Surgical Nursing Practice and Arthritis Health Professions Association. Atlanta, GA: Arthritis Foundation; 1983.
7. Moncur C. Physical therapist competencies in rheumatology. Phys Ther 1985;65: 1365–1372.
8. Caruso LA. Role and functions of occupational therapy in the management of patients with rheumatic diseases. Am J Occup Ther 1986;40:825–829.
9. Association of Rheumatology Health Professionals. Briefing Papers. Available at http://rheumatology.org/arhp/briefing/index.asp?aud=rhp.
10. American College of Rheumatology and Association of Rheumatology Health Professionals. Multidisciplinary care for patients with rheumatic and musculoskeletal diseases. Available at http://rheumatology.org/arhp/position.asp?aud=rhp.
11. Haag D. Personal communication. December 2008.
12. Moncur C. Personal communication. November 2008.
13. Clark. B Personal communication. November 2008.

# Chapter 4

# The Research and Education Foundation (REF)

James R. O'Dell

*University of Nebraska Medical Center, Department of Internal Medicine, Nebraska Medical Center, Omaha, NE*

It has been said that the American College of Rheumatology (ACR) is about the present and that the Research and Education Foundation (REF) is about the future of rheumatology. This 75th anniversary of the ACR gives us a chance to reflect on the much shorter history of the REF and perhaps dream about a vision for the "future of rheumatology."

The REF was established in 1985 as a natural consequence of the ACR splitting from the Arthritis Foundation. With the ACR established as a 501(c)6 organization, it was the foresight of Bill Kelley and many others that an affiliated organization that could accept charitable contributions would be important. Therefore, the REF, a 501(c)3 organization, was born. In its early years, a modest portfolio of programs was overseen by the ACR officers themselves. The REF's first annual report was published just 15 years ago in 1993, and it listed accomplishments that included a doubling of its annual support from $230,000 to $500,000 for 1993. At that time, the REF funded three main projects: Medical Student Summer Research Program, ACR Arthritis Investigator Award, and the Physician Scientist Development Award. Like all successful organizations, the REF has benefited from visionary leadership. The REF's

**TABLE 4.1   REF Presidents**

| Year | REF President |
|------|---------------|
| 1991–1992 | Arthur L. Weaver, MD (ACR Secretary) |
| 1993–1994 | Ronald L. Kaufman, MD (ACR Secretary) |
| 1995–1999 | Daniel Wallace, MD |
| 2000–2001 | Stanley B. Cohen, MD |
| 2002–2003 | Joseph Golbus, MD |
| 2004–2005 | Michael H. Weisman, MD |
| 2006–2007 | James R. O'Dell, MD |
| 2008–2009 | Leslie Crofford, MD |

first president, who was separate from ACR officers, was Dan Wallace who served from 1996 to 1999 (Table 4.1).

The modern-day REF really began to take shape at the turn of the century when, through the wisdom of Stan Cohen and many others, the Industrial Round Table (IRT) was created. Through the unrestricted resources made available from our industry partners who have shared our vision of a better rheumatological community, the REF has matured. We will forever be grateful for the nine founding IRT members (Amgen, Aventis, Centocor, Eli Lilly, Immunex, Knoll, Merck, Pharmacia, and Wyeth-Ayerst) and for all the other companies who have become IRT partners. Rheumatology in the United States certainly has a brighter present and future because of them.

With the income from the IRT, the REF was able to begin a phase of substantial expansion of its portfolio of grants (Table 4.2). With these resources available, it was critically important for the REF to develop a vision for what it wanted to be and for what central core values it would have. Guided by the first REF Strategic Plan in 2001, the core values of support for the training of rheumatologists and support for research

**TABLE 4.2   REF Program Services (Research, Education, Within Our Reach)**

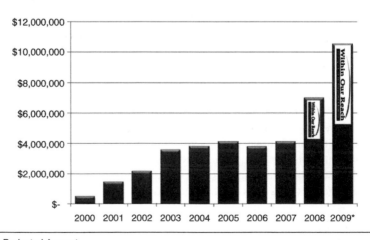

*FY 2009—Budgeted Amount

career development of rheumatologists and health professionals began to take shape. A central pillar of the first strategic plan was to increase the numbers of rheumatology fellows to 325 by the year 2006 and to have 70% of them stay in the United States after completion of their training. This latter stipulation was put in place to be consistent with the REF goal to support and address the severe shortage of rheumatologists in this country. This lofty goal was felt by many to be impossible because, at that time, only about 200 fellows were in training and only 35% of them were graduates of U.S. medical schools. In fact, the goal was reached and exceeded in 2005, a year ahead of schedule. Because even this number may not enough to meet the need for rheumatologists in this country, the REF is now in the process of setting a new, higher goal.

The second strategic plan was developed in 2005 to cover the years 2006–2010. Again, the REF established several bold goals: Expand core programs by 10% per year, create a $25 million endowment to support core programs in perpetuity, establish the Within Our Reach campaign to raise and spend $30 million for the best rheumatoid arthritis research, and raise $1 million per year from nonindustry sources. With this plan, the REF was venturing into the fundraising for specific targeted diseases, and therefore, the first pillar of this plan, the expansion of our core programs and creation of the endowment for their support, was critical to make it absolutely clear that the core values of the REF would remain: support for training of rheumatologists and support for research career development. The REF is on target to fund the endowment fully by 2010 and has at the same time expanded the core programs, including the RSDA (Research Scientist Development Award) program and rheumatology fellowship training awards, by 10% per year.

The Within Our Reach campaign has been nothing short of remarkable, in terms of both the fundraising and the fund giving. The importance of the lead ACR Pinnacle gift ($5 million), which dramatically demonstrated the commitment of the College, cannot be overemphasized. The goals of this campaign were multifactorial: Stimulate research for one of our core diseases, RA, which is drastically underfunded; support our academic training centers with these research funds so they will be available to train the next generation of rheumatologists; engage our membership in this effort specifically and the REF generally; and begin to tap into the vast donor potential that we have in our patients. This effort has clearly touched a nerve in the research community with the number (225) and quality of grants received in the first three cycles, and the accolades of the research community, both investigators and funding agencies (National Institutes of Health [NIH] and others), are remarkable. Importantly, this campaign has energized a large group of our practitioners (Ambassadors and Diplomats) who had not previously been engaged in REF activities, and they in turn have engaged their research-minded patients. For the REF to remain successful in the long term, active involvement from both of these groups will be critical. To date, success in all of the goals of the campaign has occurred; $25 million has been raised, and $12 million of research grants have been funded in the first two cycles.

Many of our industry partners have shared in our vision even above and beyond their IRT membership. They have supported programs that helped us achieve funding levels for PSDAs (Centocor), fellowship training awards (Amgen/Wyeth), pediatric visiting professor programs (Amgen), and programs to attract medical students and residents into rheumatology (Abbott) that would not have been otherwise possible. Many of our industry sponsors have also stepped up to the plate to help us with the Within Our Reach campaign, including Pinnacle Donors [Abbott, BMS (Bristol-Myers Squibb), and UCB].

Throughout its history, the REF has been extremely proud of the fact that, on average, 90% of the funds that are raised go directly to grantees. This puts the REF in select company as a charitable organization and makes it an attractive place for members and grateful patients to get the most for their money. In fact, the REF itself has underwritten the cost of the Within Our Reach campaign, so that every dollar donated in that campaign goes directly to grantees.

The REF, with a tremendous growth spurt in the last several years (Table 4.2), has now reached adolescence. Throughout its early years, the REF has dared to dream big. As it matures into adulthood, we hope to continue to support the core mission and to dream even bigger. Increased support by members and patients will be critical. As ACR members themselves mature, we hope and expect them to support the REF with planned giving so that we can grow our programs and do so with a broader support base.

# Chapter 5

# Pediatric Rheumatology: A Personal History

James T. Cassidy

*University of Missouri HSC, Department of Child Health, Columbia, MO*

Are we there yet? Perhaps. Certainly, much progress has occurred in the last 48 years. When I joined the American College of Rheumatology (ACR) in the late 1950s, our meetings were small compared with today, which consisted of about 800 members in a good year, and pediatric papers were relatively rare. My first paper in 1961 was the only one on that part of the program. Later, the need for presentation of data related to children increased, and by 1969, a pediatric concurrent session became an integral part of the meetings.

## 5.1 COMMITTEE ON CLASSIFICATION OF JUVENILE RHEUMATOID ARTHRITIS

Our progress in pediatric rheumatology was aided by the appointment in 1964 by President Marian Ropes of a committee to study the classification of juvenile rheumatoid arthritis. After decades of testing and publication of many preliminary criteria, the final report was issued in 1986 [1]. The Cincinnati Data Base was the basis of the final statistical analysis with the Arthritis, Rheumatism, Aging and Medical Information System (ARAMIS) computation system based at Stanford with J. Fries and A. Masi (Figure 5.1).

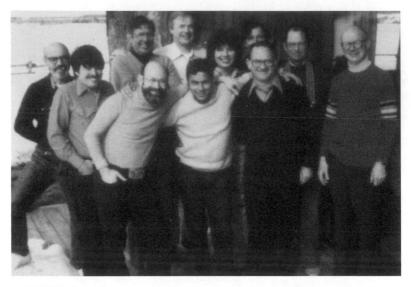

**FIGURE 5.1.** *Committee on Classification of JRA. Jackson Hole, Wyoming.*

## 5.2   PEDIATRIC COUNCIL

The first conjoint meeting on pediatrics came in 1972 in conjunction with orthopaedic surgeons in Glen Cove, New York. It certainly seemed that our small group of pediatric rheumatologists was on its way. Then, in 1975, a Pediatric Council was constituted to be a guiding force for our activities. Its membership was to include an orderly process of adding a new member and electing a chair as each old member retired. The Council met the next year in Park City, Utah, with an objective to plan an international meeting devoted to pediatric rheumatology. At that time, Lynn Bonfiglio became our staff liaison and stayed with our activities for many years. At the subsequent meeting in 1976, the attendance was approximately 187 members, with Barbara Ansell and Eric Bywaters and members of the Executive Committee of the ACR present (Figure 5.2). In this year, 123 papers were presented and discussed. These papers were printed in a supplement of *Arthritis and Rheumatism* and were published as a book whose review was coordinated by Jane Schaller and Virgil Hanson. This "Proceedings of the First ARA Conference on the Rheumatic Diseases of Childhood [2]" became the interim reference source. Other personal surveys were published by Barbara Ansell, Earl Brewer on juvenile rheumatoid arthritis (JRA), and Jerry Jacobs, the last two in second editions. In 1982, the *Textbook of Pediatric Rheumatology* was published. Ross Petty was added as an editor with the second edition. This book is now in its fifth edition, which was published in 2005, with an editorial board that includes Ron Laxer and Carol Lindsley, and a sixth edition is to be released in 2010.

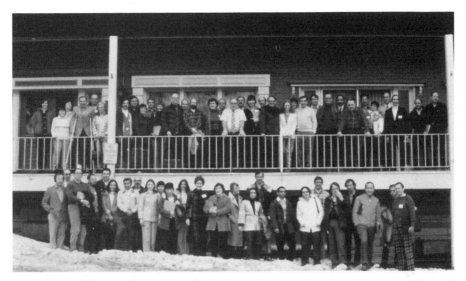

FIGURE 5.2. *Participants and guests at the First Park City Conference on the Rheumatic Diseases of Children, March 22–25, 1976.*

## 5.3 SECTION OF RHEUMATOLOGY COMMITTEE

The American Academy of Pediatrics (AAP), under the guidance of Earl Brewer, formed a Section of Rheumatology Committee in 1981. This section began to meet later with the ACR annually and established two awards when Charles Spencer was Chair. In addition, a visiting professor program was instituted, in which three medical schools without pediatric rheumatology were visited each year for 3 to 5 days. The program has been a success, and its support is now endowed. The Section also assumed responsibility for the next two Park City meetings. Subsequently, the ACR took over the subsequent meetings; the last one was at the Keystone Resort in 2008.

## 5.4 AMERICAN JUVENILE ARTHRITIS ORGANIZATION

The Arthritis Foundation established the American Juvenile Arthritis Organization, with a meeting of the initial Executive Committee in Cleveland in 1981; two pediatric members of the ACR were present: Joseph Levinson and me. This was the only organization that included lay representatives and patients along with pediatric rheumatologists. The first meeting was held in Colorado in the summer of 1984 at the Keystone Resort.

## 5.5 PEDIATRIC RHEUMATOLOGY BOARDS

In 1988, three members of the ACR, including Earl Brewer and Deborah Kredich, met at the headquarters of the AAP to complete an application for a Subboard of Pediatric

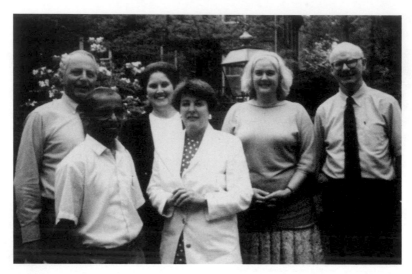

**FIGURE 5.3.** Members of the first Subboard of Pediatric Rheumatology, Chapel Hill, North Carolina.

Rheumatology in the American Board of Pediatrics. The application was accepted without objection at a subsequent meeting of the American Board of Medical Specialties. The subboard was constituted in 1990 with Kredich as Chair (Figure 5.3). Our initiative would not have been successful except for the solid support of Tim Oliver. The *Textbook* served as a compendium to the scope of the field for the first examination in 1995.

## 5.6 BLUE RIBBON COMMITTEE

During a review of the activities of the ACR, we were asked in 1997 to form a Blue Ribbon Committee to survey progress that had been made in pediatric rheumatology and to determine what was still necessary for sustainable growth [3]. This report was discussed and adopted by the ACR in 1999. Three problems highlighted were the poor representation of our specialty geographically, the linked lack of representation in our medical schools, and the small number of fellows in training. Although the number of fellows in training has improved recently to approximately 65, this observation may be somewhat misleading, as the number in each of the 3 years decreases each year and those held by international medical graduates is substantial. We have insufficient knowledge how many of those trainees will decide to remain in this country. But during these years, a tremendous increase in enthusiasm has occurred for our specialty among pediatric house officers. At the time of the first Park City meeting, there were only about 27 pediatric rheumatologists of differing backgrounds and training in 17 medical schools [4]. These numbers have now increased to over 237 in 76 centers as fellowships moved beyond Ann Arbor, Boston, Cincinnati, Houston, Los Angeles, New York, and Seattle to 26 approved programs of training.

## 5.7 SURGEON GENERAL'S REPORT

In June 1986, the Surgeon General C. Everett Koop, in recognition of problems in the care of children with special health care needs, including the large number of those with the rheumatic diseases, issued his Surgeon General's Report on Children with Special Health Care Needs [5] after a 3-day meeting in Houston that emphasized family-centered, community-based, coordinated care in the long-term follow-up of these children. Subsequently, many outreach centers were established from pediatric rheumatology programs to carry out the mandate of this report, which was sponsored by the Office of Maternal and Child Health. After approximately a decade, this program was phased out, but the knowledge gained had become an integral element of the care of a rheumatic child, with the family as the center point of coordination and the rheumatology clinic periodically instituting changes in therapy.

## 5.8 PEDIATRIC RHEUMATOLOGY COLLABORATIVE CLINICS

Another group of clinical investigators who have played an important role in our progress during these formative years was the Pediatric Rheumatology Collaborative Clinics, which were formed in 1970 under the direction of Brewer. This group has supervised several studies of therapy for JRA. Daniel Lovell is now chair of this organization. The design and analysis of results of each study has been under the direction of Edward Giannini until 2008. Recently, a second group has been formed to investigate newer modalities of treatment, which is the Childhood Arthritis and Rheumatology Research Alliance.

So I need to answer the question: Are we there yet? Fortunately, the end point is not clearly defined, but I can confidently say that we have made enormous progress that would not have been possible two or three decades earlier. Finally, it is reassuring to note that nine ACR awards of distinction have been given to our members from 2002 to 2008. Yes, we are getting there!

## REFERENCES

1. Cassidy JT, Levinson JE, Bass JC,et al. A study of classification criteria for a diagnosis of juvenile rheumatoid arthritis. Arthritis Rheum 1986;29:274–278.
2. Schaller JG, Hanson V. Proceedings of the First ARA Conference on the Rheumatic Diseases of Childhood. Arthritis Rheum 1977;20:145–636.
3. American College of Rheumatology Blue Ribbon Committee for Academic Pediatric Rheumatology. The future status of pediatric rheumatology in the United States: Strategic planning for the year 2000. Arthritis Rheum 2000;43:239–242.
4. Cassidy JT. Pediatric rheumatology: Fellowship training requirements and survey of specialty needs. Rheum Dis Clin N Am 1987;13:169–173.
5. Koop CE. Children with special health care needs. Campaign '87. U.S. Department of Health and Human Services. Public Health Service. 1987:3–40.

Chapter *6*

# The ACR: A Worldwide Organization

**Sherine E. Gabriel**

*Health Sciences Research, Mayo Clinic, Rochester, MN*

As I contemplated preparing this chapter over the past several weeks, one question kept recurring to me: What does it mean to be a worldwide organization? The more I investigated and considered this question, the clearer the answer became with respect to the American College of Rheumatology (ACR). A truly worldwide organization takes a global view of its vision, mission, and strategies. A truly worldwide organization also embraces its role as a responsible world citizen. As I hope you will agree after reading the brief comments below, the ACR has clearly demonstrated its commitment to continue to grow as a worldwide organization.

The commitment of the ACR to maintaining and enhancing an international perspective begins with its membership. The ACR has always encouraged and nurtured a large international membership. In fact, international membership (including fellows, members, and international trainees) has increased nearly 21% since 1998. In addition, the percentage of international members, as a proportion of total membership, has also increased over the past decade. International members enjoy all the privileges of American members and are encouraged to participate in all activities of the college. Whether it is a scientific discussion or a policy debate, the ACR has always taken the view that varied viewpoints enrich the dialog and improve the final outcome.

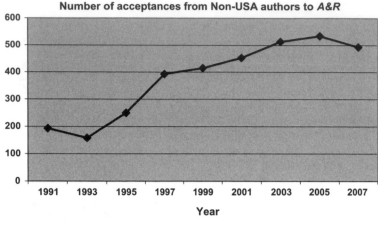

FIGURE 6.1.

Our academic activities have also taken on an increasingly international perspective. The ACR Annual Meeting has always been the meeting place for the international rheumatology community. Indeed, in recent years the proportion of international attendees has increased significantly. Also, the number of acceptances to *Arthritis & Rheumatism* from international authors has risen rather dramatically since 1991 (see Figure 6.1).

As summarized in the editorial, "Rheumatology gone global, [1]" the ACR has recently stepped up its international scientific activities even more. The ACR has been discussing collaboration with the European League Against Rheumatism (EULAR) for over 3 years, and the first fruits of this landmark achievement are now blossoming. Aletaha and colleagues [2–5] from Europe and North America developed recommendations on reporting disease activity in clinical trials of patients with rheumatoid arthritis (RA). This chapter (along with the accompanying editorial) were published simultaneously in both the ACR and the EULAR journals. Thus, this international team of experts jointly developed and published an important scientific manuscript that will serve as a guide for investigators worldwide in reporting disease activity in RA clinical trials.

This was no small feat!! Although global collaboration is nothing new in science, bringing two organizations (and their bureaucracies) together around a scientific goal was a challenge. However, the collaboration progressed because both organizations shared a common purpose: *to develop the best science and improve care for rheumatic disease patients worldwide.* The ACR and EULAR also agreed early on three guiding principles to undergird the relationship. The first principle is transparency, which is achieved through reciprocal membership on relevant committees and joint decision making. The second principle is proactive joint planning for future project ideas, and the final principle is a commitment to collaborate and not compete. With a common purpose and agreed on guiding principles, these two organizations will build what promises to be a long and productive collaboration.

The collaboration focuses on concrete projects in two areas. The first area is guidance on how to report results from trials in RA patients. Rheumatology trials are increasingly global in their scope, and trialists worldwide need a common set of guidelines to follow. The ACR recognizes that expertise for conducting the best trials is international. Thus, although regulatory agencies can have slightly different requirements, bringing together EULAR and ACR for collaboration in this area was natural. The second area of collaboration focuses on measurement in rheumatology clinical research. Valid classification and response criteria are critical for conducting high-quality research in rheumatology. The data sets and experience for developing and validating these criteria sets are global. This collaboration will enable the ACR, together with EULAR, to advance the clinical, educational, and research endeavors of rheumatologists not only in North America but all over the world.

A central motivation underlying the growing interest in international collaboration in rheumatology is the emerging evidence of major inequities in health care for rheumatic and other chronic diseases, both within and among countries. The ACR recognizes its responsibility to help advance rheumatology in areas of the world that suffer disproportionately from such inequities. Together with leaders of African League Against Rheumatism (AFLAR), Asia Pacific League Against Rheumatism (APLAR), and Pan American League Against Rheumatism (PANLAR), and in partnership with EULAR, the ACR led an initiative to restructure and reinvigorate the International League of Associations for Rheumatology (ILAR). The new ILAR now has a more focused mission to advance rheumatology in developing countries. The ACR provides administrative and management support to the new ILAR at no charge. The new ILAR Executive Committee consists of the Presidents and Presidents–Elect of ACR, AFLAR, APLAR, EULAR, and PANLAR. The collaboration among the leaders of these international organizations demonstrates a renewed commitment to support programs that advance the clinical practice and education of rheumatology in countries in which an exceptional need exists.

I have had the privilege of participating in the ILAR Executive Committee meetings and have personally witnessed the genuine enthusiasm and deep commitment to advance rheumatology in the neediest countries of the world. ILAR's newly formed Executive Committee has now endorsed the ILAR mission, resolved governance issues, and launched a new program to fund ILAR projects aimed at improving rheumatology care in countries represented by the PANLAR, APLAR, and AFLAR leagues. To date, this program has been enthusiastically received. Because the unexpectedly large number of projects submitted exceeded the funds available, this international alliance has committed to work together to identify additional funding sources. This collaborative initiative will have a positive impact on rheumatology patient care in some of the neediest areas of the world.

As noted, a truly worldwide organization takes a global view of its vision, mission, and strategies. The ACR recognizes that full realization of its potential requires contributing to, learning from, and collaborating with rheumatology colleagues all over the world. This is exemplified by the increasing emphasis on international membership and publication in ACR journals, as well as on ongoing efforts to ensure that the ACR national scientific meeting continues to be the gathering place for the international rheumatology community. A truly worldwide organization also embraces its role as a responsible world citizen. In leading the effort to create a renewed ILAR, the ACR has embraced this responsibility. The new ILAR will work to break down the geographic barriers that superficially divide the rheumatology community and to advance progress toward our common goal of creating a strong and unified global specialty and reducing health inequality worldwide. Through its collaboration with EULAR, the ACR is accelerating the development of scientifically rigorous classification and response criteria. Together, these activities demonstrate that the ACR has truly lived up to its vision of becoming a worldwide organization.

Reflecting on the past 75 years of evolution of the ACR, which are chronicled in this commemorative book, it is evident that the ACR has grown from a small national organization to an organization with worldwide membership, a world vision, and worldwide influence in rheumatology In the years to come, I believe we will witness an even greater international focus and presence for the ACR.

## REFERENCES

1. Solomon DH, Tyndall A, Gabriel SE, Dougados M. Rheumatology gone global. Ann Rheum Dis 2008;67:1357.
2. Aletaha D, Landewe R, Karonitsch T, et al. Reporting disease activity in clinical trials of patients with rheumatoid arthritis: EULAR/ACR collaborative recommendations. Arthritis Rheum 2008;59:1371–1377.
3. Karonitsch T, Aletaha D, Boers M, et al. Methods of deriving EULAR/ACR recommendations on reporting disease activity in clinical trials of patients with rheumatoid arthritis. Ann Rheum Dis 2008;67:1365–1373.
4. Aletaha D, Landewe R, Karonitsch T, et al. Reporting disease activity in clinical trials of patients with rheumatoid arthritis: EULAR/ACR collaborative recommendations. Ann Rheum Dis 2008;67:1360–1364.
5. Aletaha D, Funovits J, Smolen JS. The importance of reporting disease activity states in rheumatoid arthritis clinical trials. Arthritis Rheum 2008;58:2622–2631.

# Chapter 7

# The Relationship Between the ACR and the EULAR

**Josef S. Smolen**

*Krankenhaus Lainz, 2nd Department of Medicine, Vienna, Austria*

**Maxime Dougados**

*Department of Rheumatology, Cochin Hospital Medical Faculty, Descartes University, Paris, France*

**David A. Fox**

*Division of Rheumatology, Department of Internal Medicine, University of Michigan, Ann Arbor, MI*

**Ferdinand C. Breedveld**

*Leiden University Medical School, Leiden, the Netherlands*

Commemorative books provide a unique opportunity to appraise the past, to learn from that history, and to contemplate and advance the future. It is, therefore, a dual pleasure for us to write this chapter. The first pleasure relates to the occasion of conveying sincere congratulations to the American College of Rheumatology (ACR) on its jubilee in this special and enduring way. The second pleasure concerns the chance to review the evolution of a fruitful collaboration between two major organizations in rheumatology, which has arisen during the past few years.

## 7.1   DIFFERENCES AND SIMILARITIES

Let us briefly consider the two organizations. The European League Against Rheumatism (EULAR) is a much younger organization than the ACR, as it was founded in 1947 and thus just recently celebrated its 50th anniversary. The ACR and EULAR have both common as well as distinct characteristics and goals. The major difference relates to the constituencies. Although the ACR is an organization of individual members, EULAR's membership consists of national societies. Also, ACR members are primarily rheumatologists, either trained or in training, as well as allied rheumatology health professionals; in contrast, EULAR's members are national rheumatologic ("scientific") societies as well as national patient organizations ("Social Leagues"). Consequently, at EULAR's General Assembly, every country has two votes, one representing the patient organizations and another one for the rheumatological societies. Furthermore, one Vice President of the EULAR represents European allied health professionals. Thus, EULAR may be recognized as an equivalent of three U.S. associations, the ACR, the Arthritis Foundation, and the ARHP, albeit as an umbrella organization of respective national societies or groups.

Because health care in Europe is a national effort, the EULAR does not have to deal with many issues, such as reimbursement and health care policy, which the ACR handles for its membership. Also, the ACR's negotiating partners include government agencies and the Congress of the United States, whereas EULAR's activities focus on the European Commission headed in Brussels. Because the structure of the European Union with its Commission, Council, and Parliament is complex, the activities of EULAR are complicated by the need to act in multiple and multilateral ways, in Brussels as well as on the various national levels. Moreover, those European countries that are not member states of the European Union are also represented by EULAR.

However, the two organizations, share many similarities, which are reflected in their mission statements (Table 7.1) [1,2]. Of particular importance, both organizations are intensively involved in issues of training as well as in the creation of educational material. The ACR engages in these activities through its Research and Education Foundation (REF), its standing committees such as the Committee on Education, as well as the activities of special task forces. The EULAR pursues these goals via its Standing Committee on Education, which organizes courses (clinical, sonography, and many others) and now offers an online course on rheumatic diseases. Education is likely to be an area of intense collaboration between ACR and EULAR in the future, because pertinent information about the pathogenesis and diagnosis of musculoskeletal disorders is similar, if not identical, worldwide.

## 7.2   COMMON ACTIVITIES

Another similarity between the activities of ACR and EULAR is the development of guidance documents on clinical aspects of rheumatology. These documents concern

TABLE 7.1  Mission Statements of the ACR and the EULAR

| Mission Statement of the ACR [1] | Mission Statement of the EULAR [2] |
| --- | --- |
| The ACR is an organization of and for physicians, health professionals, and scientists that advances rheumatology through programs of education, research, advocacy and practice support that foster excellence in the care of people with or at risk for arthritis and rheumatic and musculoskeletal diseases. | The European League Against Rheumatism (EULAR) is the organisation which represents the patient, health professional and scientific societies of rheumatology of all the European nations.<br><br>The aims of EULAR are to reduce the burden of rheumatic diseases on the individual and society and to improve the treatment, prevention and rehabilitation of musculoskeletal diseases.<br><br>To this end, EULAR fosters excellence in education and research in the field of rheumatology. It promotes the translation of research advances into daily care and fights for the recognition of the needs of people with musculoskeletal diseases by the governing bodies in Europe. |

criteria for diagnosis, assessment of disease activity, and measurement parameters for clinical research studies, as well as recommendations for management or follow-up strategies. In the ACR, these strategies are created by task forces or by solicitation of proposals for work on particular topics through the Quality of Care Committee. For EULAR, this process is managed by the Standing Committee on Clinical Affairs (ESCCA); usually, EULAR members make proposals for the development of particular guidance documents to the Standing Committees consistent with standard operating procedures [3]. To avoid duplication of work or contradictory sets of criteria, it is in this area that collaborative efforts have most recently developed between ACR and EULAR. Indeed, the results of a first common EULAR/ACR activity on recommendations for clinical trial reporting have recently been published [4,5].

Currently, several other joint ventures are developing, which include criteria for the classification of rheumatoid arthritis, dermato-polymyositis and polymyalgia rheumatica; criteria for remission in rheumatoid arthritis; gout responder criteria; and recommendations for considering the diagnosis of systemic vasculitis. Thus, the ACR and EULAR have embarked on a common path that hopefully will be highly successful. To facilitate such activities, the EULAR has created the position of a liaison to the ACR as a nonvoting member of the EULAR Executive Committee. Also, there is mutual participation of representatives of each organization at the EULAR Standing Committee, ACR Quality of Care Committee, and ACR Criteria Subcommittee meetings. Operating procedures for these activities have recently been formulated [6].

An additional commonality is that both ACR and EULAR organize annual congresses, each attended by more than 10,000 participants, with a major focus on advances in the basic and clinical sciences relevant to the rheumatic diseases and on state-of-art clinical and educational information. Indeed, these two meetings today constitute global events, surpassing any other similar activity. Because congresses of the International League of Associations for Rheumatology (ILAR) have ceased, the global scope of the ACR and EULAR meetings has become especially important. These two meetings are regarded as complementary by both organizations because, even in a time frame of a few months, significant new information can develop and be disseminated in a timely manner, and the participants in the two meetings are largely nonoverlapping. Thus, these two conferences provide a service to the broad international constituency connected to rheumatology. Importantly, abstracts submitted to one meeting can also be presented at the other conference, fostering the widest exchange of novel data. The committees that plan these meetings include members representative of the other organization. For several years, it is at these two conferences where the members of the ACR and EULAR Executive Committees meet in a friendly and collaborative atmosphere to discuss new information and joint activities.

Finally, both organizations have their "own" journals, *Arthritis & Rheumatism (A&R)* and *Annals of the Rheumatic Diseases (ARD)*. Whereas *A&R* has been the official ACR journal for many decades, EULAR has only acquired *ARD*—a journal that is actually much older than *A&R*—during the last decade. Today, these journals are listed as numbers 1 and 2 in the citation indices on impact factor (IF), which represents their leadership in providing research advances and timely education for the field of rheumatology.

Does competition exist between the two organizations? Certainly, there is interest as to how the organizations compare with respect to meeting attendance and journal impact factor. Competition can be healthy, however, and, indeed can energize organizations and their members to do their best job. Currently, the ACR and EULAR are both flourishing and highly value the goals of their common activities and the efforts of those who work together on these collaborative projects. With strong collaboration and interactions, the work of both organizations can go forward productively and synergistically.

## 7.3 LOOKING INTO THE FUTURE

So where are we heading in the future? Of course, many areas are still in need of improvement. Research insights and the evidence behind them ought to be conveyed to the practicing rheumatologist more quickly and effectively. Many new guidance documents are needed, whether produced by one or both organizations. As an example, in light of the results of some recent clinical trials in systemic lupus erythematosus (SLE) [7] and expanding on existing work done by EULAR [8,9], one could envisage a joint EULAR-ACR project on clinical trial design in this disease.

Common activities might go beyond the creation of documents. Although ACR is a North American organization and EULAR is a European organization, both are global societies. Because rheumatology is not confined to North America and Europe, ACR and EULAR may also have opportunities to embark on more global activities.

Is rheumatology developing adequately in Latin America, poorer parts of Asia, and Africa? If not, how can we assist our colleagues from the less affluent regions in the world? What can we learn from them and what they from us? How can we support their goals and needs, and how best can we interact with AFLAR, APLAR, and PANLAR? Indeed, the mission statement of ACR and the second paragraph of EULAR's mission statement (Table 7.1) are not confined to a particular region of the world and thus can be used as a basis to offer our colleagues from the less industrialized world the support they need. Aside from the responsibility to their immediate constituencies, global health in the rheumatic diseases is where EULAR and ACR may find additional common interests. In meeting this challenge, important issues will concern the mechanisms of support and its distribution, as well as the areas of rheumatology that may be targeted for investment. In fact, some of these activities are already being pursued by the newly structured ILAR, in which ACR, EULAR and other regional leagues have a common platform [10] and a shared agenda—the advancement of global health in the rheumatic diseases.

In summary, we have come a long way. The ACR and EULAR are departing from their "splendid isolation" of the past in search of common ground and engagement in activities that move the field faster and better into the future—for the sake of research and clinical medicine, for the sake of patients and health care professionals, and for the future of our field—rheumatology.

## REFERENCES

1. Mission Statement. Available: http://www.rheumatology.org/about/mission.asp?aud=pat. Accessed Dec 31, 2008.

2. EULAR Mission Statement. Available: http://www.eular.org/index.cfm?framePage=/eular_mission_statement.cfm Accessed December 31, 2008.

3. Dougados M, Betteridge N, Burmester GR, et al. EULAR standardised operating procedures for the elaboration, evaluation, dissemination, and implementation of recommendations endorsed by the EULAR standing committees. Ann Rheum Dis 2004;63:1172–1176.

4. Aletaha D, Landewe R, Karonitsch T, et al. Reporting disease activity in clinical trials of patients with rheumatoid arthritis: EULAR/ACR collaborative recommendations. Ann Rheum Dis 2008;67:1360–1364.

5. Aletaha D, Landewe R, Karonitsch T, et al. Reporting disease activity in clinical trials of patients with rheumatoid arthritis: EULAR/ACR collaborative recommendations. Arthritis Rheum 2008;59:1371–1377.

6. EULAR/ACR Collaborative Projects: Standard Operating Procedures. Available: http://www.eular.org/myUploadData/files/SOP%20-%20EULAR-ACR%20collaborative%20projects%20-%20Oct%202008.pdf. Accessed Jan 2, 2009.

7. Isenberg D, Gordon C, Merrill J, et al. New therapies in systemic lupus erythematosus—trials, troubles and tribulations. . . . working towards a solution. Lupus 2008;17:967–970.

8. Gordon C, Bertsias GK, Ioannidis JP, et al. EULAR recommendations for points to consider in conducting clinical trials in systemic lupus erythematosus (SLE). Ann Rheum Dis 2008;6:1656–1662.

9. Bertsias GK, Ioannidis JP, Boletis J, et al. Evidence for selection of end-points for clinical trials in systemic lupus erytematosus (SLE): a systematic literature review. Report of a Task Force of the EULAR Standing Committee for International Clinical Studies Including Therapeutics (ESCISIT). Ann Rheum Dis 2008.

10. ILAR Mission Statement. Available: http://www ilar org/mission-statement asp 2009.

*Chapter* 8

---

# *Scientific Publications*

**Michael D. Lockshin**

*Hospital for Special Surgery-Cornell, New York, NY*

This discussion of "scientific publications" considers the history of *Arthritis & Rheumatism* (*A&R*) and the future of rheumatology publication.

## 8.1  HISTORY

In the first issue of *A&R* (Figure 8.1), Robert M. Stecher described the history of this journal. A meeting in Paris in April 1925 concluded with a call for an international rheumatology committee, which was established and led to the development of national organizations. These organizations developed their own journals. The first rheumatology journal was *Acta Rheumatologica*, which was a Scandinavian journal first published (in English) in 1929 (Table 8.1). Other European and South American journals followed. The American Rheumatism Association (later named the American College of Rheumatology [ACR]) began in 1934 but did not establish its own journal, *A&R*, until 1958. *Arthritis Care & Research (AC&R)* was first a journal of the Association of Rheumatology Health Professionals section of the Arthritis Foundation (from 1988) and became part of *A&R* in 2001.

---

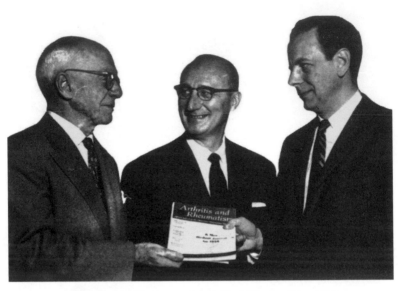

**FIGURE 8.1.** *First issue of Arthritis & Rheumatism; 1958.*

## 8.2   STATISTICS REGARDING A&R

In 2008, 79% of *A&R*'s papers concerned studies on human subjects, whereas the rest involved animals; 57% were basic science topics, and the rest were clinical. Papers concern all rheumatological diseases; rheumatoid arthritis and osteoarthritis are the

**TABLE 8.1   Founding Dates of Rheumatology Journals and Reviews, as Cited by Stecher or as Identified from Contemporary Websites (Search October 5, 2008); Journals Introduced after 1974 are not Included**

| Journal | Year | Language |
|---|---|---|
| *Acta Rheumatologica* | 1929 | English |
| *Primer on Rheumatism (reviews)* | 1932 or 1934[*] | English |
| *Revue du Rhumatisme* | 1934 | French |
| *Revista Argentina de Reumatologia* | 1936 | Spanish |
| *Archivos Argentinos de Reumatologia* | 1937 | Spanish |
| *Rheumatism Reviews (reviews)* | 1937 | English |
| *Zeitschrift für Rheumatologie* | 1938 | German |
| *Rheumatism (London) (reviews)* | 1938 | English |
| *British Journal of Rheumatism* | 1938 | English |
| *Bulletin of American Rheumatism Assoc (reviews)* | 1938 | English |
| *Annals of Rheumatic Diseases* | 1939 | English |
| *Reumatismo* | 1949 | Italian |
| **Arthritis & Rheumatism** | **1958** | **English** |
| *Revista Brasileira de Reumatologia* | 1959 | Portuguese |
| *Scandinavian Journal of Rheumatology* | 1972 | English |
| *Revista Española de Reumatologia* | 1974 | Spanish |
| *Journal of Rheumatology* | 1974 | English |

[*]Different years depend on whether the initial format is considered to be a separate journal.

**TABLE 8.2   Articles Published January 1–September 30, 2008, on Selected Topics, Identified by Keywords "Rheumatoid," "Osteoarthritis," "Lupus," or "Cartilage" in Title, as Listed on the Journal Website on October 5, 2008, at these Websites. http://www.rheumatology.org/publications/ar/index.asp, http://content.nejm.org/, http://jama.ama-assn.org/, http://www.nature.com/**

| Journal | RA | OA | SLE | Cartilage |
|---|---|---|---|---|
| **Arthritis &Rheumatism (monthly)** | 87 | 34 | 45 | 28 |
| New England Journal of Medicine (weekly) | 2 | 4 | 3 | 0 |
| Journal of the American Medical Association (weekly) | 0 | 0 | 0 | 0 |
| Nature/Nature Med (weekly/monthly) | 8 | 2 | 4 | 11 |

most frequent. In all, 48% of published full-length papers come from the United Kingdom and Europe, 39% from the United States and Canada, 11% from Asia, and 1% from elsewhere.

To draw comparisons among rheumatology journals and among articles published in rheumatology journals, we performed keyword Internet searches on relevant anatomy, biological molecules, and processes. Basic science searches yielded many papers not of interest to rheumatologists. Disease name searches more closely approximate the content of rheumatology journals but miss some papers that describe the basic science underpinnings of rheumatology. Table 8.2 shows the results of searches of selected, widely read journals on three disease names and on one basic science topic. Table 8.3 shows similar searches performed on the National Library of Medicine's website, PubMed. Both queries show that A&R publishes many more rheumatology papers than do general medical or general science journals.

Thomson-Reuter's Impact Factor ranks the influence of journals by listing the ratio of citations (in the succeeding 2 years) to published articles (in the examined year) (i.e., citations in 2007 and 2008 to articles published in 2006). By the Impact Factor criterion, A&R is consistently the most influential rheumatology journal in the world. Google Scholar measures influence of individual articles by ranking the number of times an article has been cited or sought (clicks), which includes Internet searches. Unlike the Impact Factor, Google Scholar's rankings are not time limited: the first 50 articles listed for osteoarthritis go back to 1939, for rheumatoid arthritis to 1949, for cartilage to 1971, and for SLE to 1983. A&R articles appear in the top 50 for the each of the disease name searches in Google Scholar.

## 8.3   THE FUTURE

We anticipate changes in content, changes in readership, evolution of an all electronic journal, and globalization.

### 8.3.1   Change in Content

Topics addressed in the first issue of A&R were rehabilitation, peripheral neuropathy, the latex fixation test, salicylates, and osteoarthritis in guinea pigs. The first issue of

**TABLE 8.3  English Language Core Clinical Journals Publishing 2 or More Papers having "Rheumatoid", "Osteoarthritis", "Lupus", or "Cartilage" in the Title**

| Disease (Total Articles) | Journal | Number |
|---|---|---|
| Rheumatoid arthritis (64) | **Arthritis &Rheumatism** | 15 |
| | **Arthritis Care &Research** | 14 |
| | Rheumatology (Oxford) | 6 |
| | Archives of Internal Medicine | 3 |
| | Journal of Immunology | 2 |
| Osteoarthritis (32) | **Arthritis Care &Research** | 9 |
| | **Arthritis &Rheumatism** | 4 |
| | Rheumatology (Oxford) | 4 |
| | Journal of Bone and Joint Surgery | 3 |
| | New England Journal of Medicine | 2 |
| | Archives of Internal Medicine | 2 |
| SLE (38) | **Arthritis &Rheumatism** | 8 |
| | **Arthritis Care &Research** | 7 |
| | Rheumatology (Oxford) | 11 |
| | Journal of Immunology | 7 |
| Cartilage (64) | **Arthritis &Rheumatism** | 27 |
| | Plastic and Reconstructive Surgery | 7 |
| | Clinical Orthopedics Related Reseearch | 4 |
| | Journal of Bone and Joint Surgery | 3 |
| | Archives of Otolaryngology and Head and Neck Surgery | 3 |
| | American Journal of Roentgenology | 3 |
| | Rheumatology (Oxford) | 2 |
| | Radiology | 2 |
| | Journal of Laryngology & Otology | 2 |
| | Journal of Oral and Maxillofacial Surgery | 2 |
| | Journal of Pediatrics | 2 |

Articles for the diseases are those published in the last 90 days, according to a PubMed search done on October 5, 2008, and articles for cartilage are those published in all of 2008 (search done October 9, 2008). The website for this search was http://www.ncbi.nlm.nih.gov/sites/entrez.

*A&R*'s 51st year (2008) focused on epidemiology, biologics, randomized double-blind controlled trials, cartilage and bone biology, cytokines, and genetic studies. Science evolves; undoubtedly, the content will be much different at the 75th or 100th anniversary of this journal.

The ACR now publishes journals with different missions. Both *A&R* and *AC&R* publish clinical studies. Basic science is a major mission of *A&R*, whereas physical medicine, guidelines, and criteria papers fall within the mission of *AC&R*. *The Rheumatologist* publishes news articles, political items, and commentary. Evolving ACR policy changes will likely alter the missions of these journals in the future.

A medical journal has several core functions: to perform peer review and identify the most meritorious papers; to copyedit accepted papers for clarity and accuracy; to filter content and quality for its audience; to provide an archive; and to support its sponsoring organization financially and intellectually. Content and national origin represent missions and not core functions; the presentation format is neither a mission nor a core function.

In maintaining their core functions, future rheumatology journals could be international; they could organize themselves according to type of article (basic science, case reports, or clinical trials). The format of electronic papers might change. What we now call "journals" could be functional links, through which a reader can select articles posted on the Internet, rather than self-contained (monthly) issues. The journal would still rule on quality and content. It would still copyedit. Its financial structure and archiving methods may change.

### 8.3.2 Change in Readership

Current readers of the print journal are mostly physicians and scientists. The Internet makes the content of journals available to patients and the public as well. Commercial and voluntary websites summarize medical literature in popular formats directed to these audiences. Whether conventional journals will alter their presentations to address these new readers is unknown.

### 8.3.3 The All-Electronic Journal

A paper journal preserves an archive; electronic journals may be unable to do so. In all other aspects—flexible graphics, ease of access, ability of readers to interact with content and with authors, and cost—electronic publication has advantage over paper. Articles can now be read on personal computers, handheld devices, web broadcasts, and electronic books.

In a future journal, an editorial board will still select submitted papers and will present a point of view. It will set quality standards for content, accuracy, and readability. Although cost and physical size limit the size of a paper journal, focus and quality criteria will limit the size of an electronic journal. A mechanism for maintaining an archive will remain.

Because its journals provide income, conversion to electronic publication could threaten the ACR's financial base. However, society-sponsored journals such as *A&R* select and recruit articles that answer the needs of interested people. In lieu of what we now call a journal, a society can provide access to such articles through computer paradigms that it provides and for which it charges fees.

### 8.3.4 Globalization

International authorship of papers published in *A&R* was almost 60% in 2007–2008. Major position papers now appear simultaneously in *AC&R* and the European League Against Rheumatism (EULAR)'s official journal, *Annals of Rheumatic Diseases*. The content of most journals is available worldwide online; international collaborations among scientists are commonplace. Science does not have national boundaries.

An argument for national identity for a journal is that national organizations sponsor and provide the journal as a service to members. Another argument is the language of publication. The first argument is one of policy, which can be changed. For the second, English is nearly universal as a scientific language, and translation is easily obtained. Even though sponsorship, copyright, and other regulatory issues need to be resolved, the flat world may render moot the continuation of national journals.

The scientific world will likely learn from other areas of commerce. Globalization of rheumatology journals will likely follow collaborative decisions made by national organization governing bodies. One can envision an international series of rheumatology journals with different audiences and different missions, the distinctions are based on content and quality but not on nationality.

Chapter *9*

# The ACR Annual Scientific Meeting

Jonathan Kay

*University of Massachusetts Medical School, Worcester, MA*

The American College of Rheumatology (ACR) Annual Scientific Meeting is the preeminent international scientific gathering of rheumatologists and is the venue where the latest clinical and scientific information relevant to the care of patients with rheumatic diseases is presented. Conducting this meeting for its members is one of the primary functions of the ACR. Over the past 75 years, this meeting has grown in both its scope and its attendance.

The first Annual Meeting of the American Association for the Study and Control of Rheumatic Diseases in Cleveland, Ohio, was attended by 75 members on June 10, 1934. Eleven scientific papers were presented at this meeting. By the next year, when the meeting was held in Atlantic City, New Jersey, on June 9, 1935, attendance had doubled to 152 members and 18 scientific papers were presented. In 1937, the American Association for the Study and Control of Rheumatic Diseases became the American Rheumatism Association. Attendance at the Annual Meeting had increased to 260 members by 1942. However, between 1943 and 1945, no annual meeting was conducted during WW II. The next Annual Meeting of the American Rheumatism Association in New York City on May 23, 1946, was attended by 285 members. Attendance subsequently grew steadily. By 1959, 1325 members attended the Annual Meeting in Washington, DC, at which 88 scientific papers were presented.

*The ACR at 75: A Diamond Jubilee*
Copyright © 2009 by John Wiley & Sons, Inc.

I first attended an Annual Meeting of the American Rheumatism Association in June 1987 at the end of my first year of fellowship training. When entering the exhibition hall, I was immediately impressed by the number of attendees at the meeting who shared my passion for rheumatology. The 1,644 members who attended the 1987 scientific meeting spanned the wide range of professional activities available to rheumatologists, from clinicians engaged in the practice of rheumatology who cared for patients on a daily basis to scientists who worked in the laboratory to elucidate the basic mechanisms of rheumatic diseases. Standing on the red carpets that cushioned the cement floor between row upon row of poster boards were the luminaries of rheumatology who I had encountered previously only by reading their publications. I was most impressed by Dr. Morris Ziff, who traveled from poster to poster and stopped at each to make a brief but helpful comment to each poster presenter. This young rheumatology trainee was captivated by the display of the range of innovation in our subspecialty.

The ACR Annual Scientific Meeting is planned by a dedicated group of volunteers who meet each January to plan the meeting for that year. These volunteers represent all aspects of rheumatology: adult and pediatric rheumatologists; laboratory scientists, health services researchers, and clinical rheumatologists; academic physicians and private practitioners. Although most of the Annual Meeting Planning Committee members work and reside in the United States, the committee also includes rheumatologists from Canada, Europe, South America, and Asia. Prior to this meeting, suggestions for sessions are solicited from the ACR membership. These suggestions, as well as evaluations by attendees of previous meetings, are reviewed by the planning committee members before their meeting.

When I first attended a meeting of the Annual Meeting Planning Committee in 1997, the meeting was held in a windowless room in an airport hotel in Atlanta. Committee members arrived on Friday evening and immediately set to work reviewing all of the sessions proposed by members. Deliberations continued late into Friday night and resumed on Saturday morning, continuing throughout the day. Meals were served in an adjacent windowless hotel meeting room. On Sunday morning, miraculously, a meeting program was shaped and finalized by the collected committee members. When next seeing sunlight on Sunday afternoon, I felt like Florestan in Beethoven's *Fidelio* emerging from darkness into the light of freedom. The tremendous accomplishment of the committee members evoked the celebratory music, in a major key, that accompanies Florestan's return to the light of the world.

In 2001, the planning meeting was moved to another airport hotel in Atlanta, where it was conducted in a room on the ground floor. The lobby outside of this meeting room was illuminated by large picture windows to allow the sunlight to shine on the Annual Meeting Planning Committee members. That year, the planning process was modified so that committee members with expertise in basic science would review proposals about basic science sessions, and those with predominantly clinical expertise would review proposals regarding clinical sessions. This division of labor hastened the process of planning the Annual Meeting and allowed for free time on Saturday evening during which the committee members had a chance to get together in a more relaxed setting. By noon on Sunday, not only was the meeting program finalized but also rooms were assigned for the various sessions.

During the tenure of Dr. Richard Furie as Annual Meeting Planning Committee chair, information technology was integrated into the planning process. Proposals for sessions were solicited from ACR members online, and the list of session proposals generated during the planning committee meeting was maintained in a database for use in planning future Continuing Medical Education meetings. Under the leadership of Dr. Brian Mandell, additional types of sessions were introduced. Novel formats, such as clinicopathologic conferences and brief clinical vignettes discussed by experts, have been extremely well received by meeting attendees.

The other major activity involved in planning the annual meeting is selection of those abstracts to be presented at the Annual Scientific Meeting. This activity is conducted by the Abstract Selection Committee, members of which are charged with selecting abstracts for poster or oral presentation and with choosing those abstracts to be highlighted in one of the three plenary abstract sessions. With the advent of targeted biologic therapies for the treatment of rheumatic diseases, the number of abstracts submitted to the Annual Scientific Meeting increased dramatically. Whereas 1,435 abstracts were submitted for consideration to be presented at the 1990 ACR Annual Scientific Meeting in Seattle, Washington, this number more than doubled to 3,023 abstracts submitted for the 2000 ACR Annual Scientific Meeting in Philadelphia, Pennsylvania.

Traditionally, the Abstract Selection Committee had been chaired by one person who had the responsibility of reading all of the abstracts and overseeing the more than 30 abstract selection subcommittees. By 2004, this job had become too enormous for one individual and it was divided between two people: a Basic Science Chair and a Clinical Chair.

Like the Annual Meeting Planning Committee, the Abstract Selection Committee meets in June or July to select the abstracts for presentation at that year's Annual Scientific Meeting. Since 2003, this process also has been facilitated by the intro-duction of information technology for abstract submission, selection, and presentation.

Once the European League Against Rheumatism (EULAR) starting holding its meeting on an annual basis in 2000, it became apparent that the eligibility guidelines for submitting abstracts to the ACR Annual Scientific Meeting needed to be reassessed. These had stated that "an abstract will not be considered if the research has been accepted for presentation at another scientific meeting or has been published or publicized in any format prior to the ACR submission deadline." To allow members of the ACR, most of whom attend only the ACR Annual Scientific Meeting, to learn first hand of the latest advances relevant to care of patients with rheumatic diseases, these eligibility guidelines were modified in 2005 to allow submission of all research. If submitted data had been presented previously at another meeting, then it was to be indicated on the abstract submission so that the Abstract Selection Committee could take this into account in reviewing the abstract. This change not only benefited the ACR members but also engendered goodwill and enhanced the relationship between the ACR and EULAR.

The ACR Annual Scientific Meeting could not take place without the tireless hard work of the ACR staff. At the first meeting that I attended in 1987, I recall vividly the image of the energetic young man bounding about the exhibition hall and communicating on a walkie talkie about logistical issues. Over the subsequent 20 years, I have gotten to know Ron Olejko, ACR Senior Director of Meetings and Conferences, whose encyclopedic knowledge of meeting venues is without equal. The indefatigable efforts of Ron and his staff contribute to the success of each meeting. Each of the planning meetings and all of the educational meetings throughout the year are run by the ACR Education Department, which is now led by Donna Hoyne, ACR Vice President for Education. Without Donna and her staff, none of the ACR educational offerings would be possible.

In this brief overview of the ACR Annual Scientific Meeting, I have certainly omitted mention of many important events and people who have contributed to making this the preeminent international assembly of rheumatologists. However, this ongoing story will continue to unfold as great progress continues to be made in the care of patients with rheumatic diseases.

# Chapter *10*

# The Role of the ACR in the Political Process

**David G. Borenstein**

*Arthritis & Rheumatism Associates, Washington, DC*

## 10.1 THE ROLE OF THE AMERICAN COLLEGE OF RHEUMATOLOGY (ACR) IN THE POLITICAL PROCESS

The First Amendment of the U.S. Constitution states "Congress shall make no law . . . abridging the freedom . . . to petition the Government for a redress of grievances". For the first 60 years of its existence, the ACR was not convinced that this fundamental right was of sufficient consequence to require the expenditure of significant time, effort, or resources. Prior to 1995, the political advocacy work of the ACR was divided between two subcommittees: a Legislative Affairs Subcommittee in the Research Council that requested increased National Institutes of Health funding for rheumatology research and a different Legislative Subcommittee in the Rheumatologic Care Council that dealt with reimbursement issues.

*The ACR at 75: A Diamond Jubilee*
Copyright © 2009 by John Wiley & Sons, Inc.

## 10.2 ESTABLISHMENT OF GOVERNMENT AFFAIRS COMMITTEE (GAC)

The need for coordination of these efforts was recognized during the strategic planning process of 1995 resulting in the establishment of a single new committee called the Committee of Legislative Affairs. The realization that the committee's role was greater than legislative issues alone resulted in the renaming of the group as the Government Affairs Committee, with Paul Katz, MD, serving as its Chairman from 1995 to 1998. Dr. Katz's efforts were directed at defining the initial scope of work of the committee. Both federal and state governmental entities were impacting the practice of rheumatology. The committee realized that the greatest benefit for the ACR was concentrating efforts with issues involving the federal government.

## 10.3 INCREASING PROCEDURAL KNOWLEDGE

In an effort to understand the regulatory and legislative processes that impacted rheumatologists, the ACR contracted with Medical Advocacy Services, Incorporated (MASI) of the American College of Physicians (ACP). MASI was the governmental lobbying organization for the ACP. MASI was able to monitor federal rules and legislative matters as they affected rheumatologists. Under the leadership of Robert Yood, MD (1998–2001), the GAC made an effort to increase the influence of the ACR in the issues of the time, such as The Patient's Bill of Rights. Through partnerships facilitated by MASI with the American Medical Association and ACP, among others, the GAC maximized our influence despite the relatively small size of our subspecialty group. These efforts increased our visibility as a group interested in advocacy among our medical colleagues.

## 10.4 INCREASING LEGISLATIVE VISIBILITY

An area of continual frustration for those involved with advocacy was the lack of recognition of government representatives, particularly legislative and regulatory entities, of the central role of rheumatology and rheumatologists as important in the care of individuals with chronic illnesses and preventable disabilities. During my tenure as chairman of GAC (2001–2004), I attempted to increase the recognition of our subspecialty by promoting the participation of our members in advocacy events on Capitol Hill. In addition, patients were invited to participate in these Congressional visits. The presence of our patients associated a human face with our requests for increased research funding and appropriate compensation for our services. The ACR also sponsored Legislative receptions that allowed members of the GAC to interact with legislators and their staff members.

## 10.5   FORMATION OF A POLITICAL ACTION COMMITTEE (PAC)

Joseph Flood, MD (2004–2007), was the chairman of GAC when two significant changes occurred. First, ACP disbanded MASI. GAC needed to decide on new representation for its lobbying efforts on Capitol Hill. GAC and the Board of Directors selected Patton Boggs, LLP, which is a law firm with professional relationships and knowledge of all branches of government, as our representative. Since its selection, Patton Boggs has served us well in presenting the ACR position on many issues, including revision of the Medicare payment system, reimbursement for dual-energy X-ray absorptiometry (DXA), and increased funding for National Institutes of Health (NIH) research. Patton Boggs gained access for our organization to those individuals who get legislation into law. This access had been unavailable to us previously. Second, GAC made the case, and the Board of Directors approved the formation of a PAC. The PAC, called Rheum PAC, under the leadership of Gary Bryant, MD, was developed to allow contributions to the election campaigns of representatives of both political parties. The donations were made to those individuals who are supportive of the positions taken by the ACR. Also during this period, as a sign of the increasing importance of advocacy for the ACR, Neil Birnbaum, MD, (Figure 10.1) who was President of the ACR in 2007, moved the May Board of Directors meeting from Chicago to Washington, DC. This schedule change allowed the Executive Committee and the Board of Directors to visit their elected representatives when Congress was in

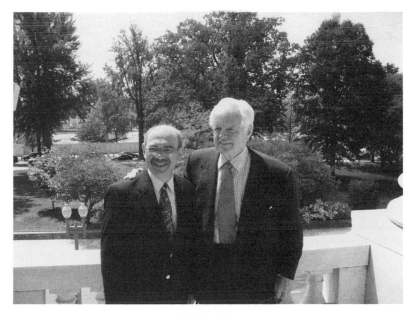

**FIGURE 10.1.**

session. The representatives of the ACR were able to express in person the importance they placed on the issues that were having an effect on health care.

## 10.6 THE ARTHRITIS ACT

The current chairman of GAC is Sharad Lakhanpal, MD (2007–2010). He has many important issues that remain to be resolved. The Arthritis Prevention, Control, and Cure Act of 2007 remains a bill and not a law. Despite efforts by the ACR and Arthritis Foundation, the Arthritis Act has not been passed by Congress. The Act would enhance rheumatic disease research by coordinating federal efforts in this area, enhance support for outreach programs to prevent and manage arthritis, and provide debt forgiveness for health professionals who enter the field of pediatric rheumatology. The bill will need to be reintroduced in the next Congress. Dr. Lakhanpal and GAC will be redoubling their efforts to get this Act passed by Congress and signed by the President into law. GAC will also be advocating for the Medicare Fracture Prevention and Osteoporosis Testing Act. This legislation has been submitted to improve reimbursement for bone mineral density testing. This legislation establishes programs with the potential to prevent fractures at a great savings of human misery and medical expenditures.

The GAC has been fortunate to have administrative staff that is essential to the success of the committee. The staff included Steven Echard, Karen Weathersbee, Aaron Johnson, Teresa Fitzgerald, Kristin Wormley, Aiken Hackett, and Tiffany Schmidt. The staff was the institutional memory for the issues that were the core purpose of the committee since its inception.

## 10.7 FUTURE OF RHEUMATOLOGY

The 75th Anniversary of the ACR coincides with a tumultuous time in the United States. Our financial crisis is real. Our health care system is failing on several levels. Although the United States spends more on each person for health care than any other country, life expectancy is ranked 45th in the world [1]. A significant proportion of health care dollars is spent on administrative misadventures to prevent the rendering of care. The reimbursement for the evaluation and treatment of patients is under constant downward pressures. Our population is aging. The need for rheumatologists will be increasing. The number of younger physicians who are choosing rheumatology is not filling the places of those older physicians who are considering retirement. The government is asking for quality in the health care it purchases. Who defines quality in medicine? Is it the government? The insurance industry? Or, preferably the ACR? Will health care reform under the new administration have the answers to these problems?

Now more than ever, political advocacy is essential to the future of our subspecialty. If we do not propose the solutions to our concerns, then others will impose them on us. Unless we have a seat at the table for these discussions, our voice will not be heard. I would hope that the next 75 years of our organization will be better than the first. This will only occur if we are diligent in making our voices heard. That is why it is crucial for our organization to be an active participant in the political process.

## REFERENCE

1. Emmanuel E.J. What cannot be said on television about health care. JAMA 2007;297:2131–2133.

# Chapter 11

# Graduate Medical Education and Training

**Dennis W. Boulware**

*Kaiser Permanente Medical Center, Honolulu, HI*

## 11.1 THE EARLY YEARS OF GRADUATE MEDICAL EDUCATION

The book, *Time to Heal: American Medical Education from the Turn of the Century to the Era of Managed Care,* by Kenneth Ludmerer, MD, PhD, professor of medicine and history at Washington University, provides a valuable framework to understand changes in medical education as rheumatology has grown as a subspecialty [1]. Prior to WW I, residency training was not commonplace, as it was assumed a medical school graduate was ready for clinical practice. That trend changed after the war as, in 1925, the American Medical Association published its first list of hospital-based residency training programs, which thereby started the GME era of modern American medicine.

One important phase in the GME era was the establishment of specialty boards that recognized the ascent of a physician to the level of a board-certified specialist (Table 11.1). The fields of internal medicine and pediatrics were relatively late adopters of specialization with the establishment of the American Board of Pediatrics (ABP) in 1933 and the American Board of Internal Medicine (ABIM) in 1936; in contrast, the American Board of Ophthalmology was the first one established in 1916.

*The ACR at 75: A Diamond Jubilee*
Copyright © 2009 by John Wiley & Sons, Inc.

**TABLE 11.1  Timeline of Important Events in GME**

1933—ABP is established
1936—ABIM is established
1972—ABIM first certifies rheumatology subspecialists
1992—ABP first certifies pediatric rheumatology subspecialists
1985—ACR Research and Education Foundation established
1987—ACGME starts adult rheumatology program accreditation
1997—ACGME starts pediatrics rheumatology program accreditation

The ABIM and ABP were even later in recognizing and awarding certification in rheumatology as a subspecialty in 1972 and 1992, respectively. Eventually, the ABIM and ABP required completion of training in an accredited fellowship program to sit for the subspecialty certification examination. It was not until 1987, however, that the Accreditation Council for Graduate Medical Education (ACGME) began accrediting training programs in adult rheumatology and in 1997 for pediatric rheumatology fellowships. This final phase of the GME era coincided with next era of modern American medicine, the research era, which began after WW II.

## 11.2  THE RESEARCH ERA

Following WW II, growth in medical research was phenomenal with estimates of national expenditures on medical research of $87 million in 1947 growing to $2.05 billion by 1966 [2]. Interest in subspecialty medicine catapulted with this research explosion, and training in research became an integral part of subspecialty fellowship training; to this day, a training program in rheumatology must contain a productive research component for accreditation. Today, medical research is entrenched in medical schools and subspecialty training programs, and despite today's difficulties in funding, medical research remains an essential component of all fellowship programs; indeed, the ACGME requires scholarship by most fellows for a program accreditation.

## 11.3  THE MANAGED CARE ERA

In 1993, heath care reform became a major topic of national discussion reflecting the campaign promise of the new American president. Although much discussion focused on enhancing the role of primary care, reform was truly targeted on cost containment and even on reduction as the growth in health care costs exceeded the growth in the Gross National Product. This growth prompted fears that health care costs would handicap national economic growth and affect global economies. In this environment, subspecialty medicine took on a negative connotation and was threatened. Applications to rheumatology fellowship programs dropped and there was concern about the quality and depth of the remaining applicant pools. Although applicant interest in rheumatology training waned, the ACGME began to require more of training programs in terms of a formal written curriculum; it also initiated plans for outcomes-based training structured on six general competencies. During one period of time, the ACGME required internal medicine fellowship programs to maintain a minimum number of enrolled fellows or risk their accreditation status. This requirement forced some programs to enroll applicants they previously would not find acceptable. The outlook seemed bleak and worsened by some projections indicating that subspecialty training and a career in rheumatology could negatively impact lifetime earning potential relative to a general internal medicine career [3]. Fortunately, this negative trend for rheumatology reversed, and applicant interest in rheumatology training rebounded strongly.

## 11.4   TODAY—A PERFECT STORM?

Many view today's health care environment as a perfect storm for training programs. Requirements for compliance and documentation, already burdensome, seem to be increasing while physician reimbursements are under constant threat of reduction. Funding for research is harder to acquire and maintain; and the accreditation requirements for training programs get more stringent and demand more effort and accountability of the faculty. Faculty in academic rheumatology training programs currently struggle as the traditional funding streams of clinical service, research, or philanthropy are reduced, while at the same time, faculty are asked to deliver more work by institutional requirements, third-party payers, funding agencies, and accrediting bodies. In this climate, faculty visualize the demands for clinical services grow with the graying of the baby boomer generation and the anticipated flood of requests for clinical services. The current situation is frustrating to many because introduction of effective therapies for diseases such as rheumatoid arthritis and the blossoming of immunology knowledge relevant to rheumatology indicate how much more could be accomplished in clinical care and discovery if only the current funding environment were less constrained.

## 11.5   THE FUTURE AND THE AMERICAN COLLEGE
## OF RHEUMATOLOGY (ACR)

The challenges to American medicine will continue in the future and may grow with the aging of America and the uncertainty of our nation's economic future. Today, faculty pressures build with the American public's growing desire for accountability from the health-care system as the cost of health care soars, the cost of higher learning rises, expenditures in research climb, and concerns of safety in the health care system ascend. Yet, at the same time, accrediting bodies are ramping up their expectations for accountability of outcomes in training. All of these converging forces adversely impact the rheumatology training programs as financial and workforce resources are typically the lowest in rheumatology divisions relative to other divisions within the departments of medicine.

As a subspecialty, we are fortunate that throughout the last two decades, the ACR anticipated these trends and developed proactive responses. When interest in subspecialty training waned in the 1990s, the ACR's Research and Education Foundation (REF) initiated programs to target medical students, residents, graduate students, and health professionals to stimulate interest in rheumatology as a profession. Also, when the ACGME announced its intent to introduce an outcomes-based accreditation system, the ACR funded retreats and forums for training program directors to prepare for these changes. At the second ACR retreat, program directors collaborated on their own set of essential competencies and outcomes, which mirrored the ACGME general competencies and assessment toolbox that were later released. The ACR was the first internal medicine subspecialty to host retreats for program directors to share experiences in improving training programs and was the first subspecialty to invite the Residency Review Committee for Internal Medicine executive director, to meet with program directors who were anticipating an accreditation site visit and advise them on potential areas of weakness that could affect program accreditation.

With the Balanced Budget Act of 1997, the funding of adult fellowship programs was jeopardized. The REF responded by offering fellowship training awards to institutions to expand rheumatology fellowship positions. Eventually, the REF offered awards to promote faculty development as clinician educators, researchers, and even reentry into academia. In the most recent fiscal year, the REF awarded more than $11 million to individuals and institutions, which established the REF as the second largest funder of research and education in rheumatology.

The future for GME training will continue to challenge training programs as no immediate relief is in sight for dwindling revenues, public demands for account-ability, and increasing documentation requirements. Although there is no agreement on solutions to these problems, rheumatology training programs should remain optimistic. First, GME will likely always feel like a challenge as even Abraham Flexner's review of all medical schools in 1910 quoted faculty who felt their multiple duties of teaching and research "encroach on a common fund of time and energy" and were at times "more or less antagonistic [4]." In the future, it is likely that our training programs will require more faculty effort in observing, assessing, and documenting trainee outcomes in acquiring clinical competence. Tools to measure these outcomes will become more refined, with developments spawned in individual programs shared and accepted through the ACR program director retreats. Research will remain integral in the fellowship programs but will likely expand to reflect a broad scope of scholarship beyond basic laboratory research.

Funding streams may never flow sufficiently to quench the faculty's thirst for resources. This situation is not a sign of greed as much as a desire for a system that fosters new knowledge, creates more effective therapies, and trains highly competent rheumatologists to meet the demands of the public. Even though current limitations on resources are frustrating and may hinder improvement in health care delivery, until a better system of funding is developed, the ACR will remain a vital resource and a beacon of promise for rheumatology to guide us through turbulent times.

# REFERENCES

1. Ludmerer KM. Time to Heal: American Medical Education from the Turn of the Century to the Era of Managed Care. New York: Oxford University Press; 1999.
2. Shannon JA. The advancement of medical research: A twenty-year view of the role of the NIH. J Med Edu 1967;42:97.
3. Prashker MJ, Meenan RF. Subspecialty training: Is it worthwhile? Ann Int Med. 1992;116:349.
4. Flexner A. Medical Education in the United States and Canada. New York: Carnegie Foundation for the Advancement of Teaching; 1910, p. 282.

# Chapter 12

# The Funding of Rheumatic Disease Research

Leslie J. Crofford

*University of Kentucky, Division of Rheumatology, Lexington, KY*

## 12.1 THE EARLY YEARS OF MEDICAL EDUCATION AND RESEARCH

My great grandfather, David M. Childers, graduated from the University of Louisville in 1892 as a Doctor of Medicine. His single year of study consisted of a series of apprenticeships with the eight faculty members affiliated with the institution, all of whom signed his diploma (one of my most prized possessions). There was no such entity as a rheumatologist to participate in his training; yet I remember being told of the respect and trust with which "Doc" Childers was viewed as he used his horse and buggy to pay house calls in rural East Texas. His only tools were his knowledge, compassion, surgical skills, and a very few medications to treat rheumatic conditions including quinine and morphine.

The concept that medical education should be undertaken only by research-oriented, university-affiliated schools rather than "trade schools" was promoted by the Flexner report of 1910 and by position of the American Medical Association. Early in the 20th century, however, medical schools had few full-time faculty, clinical practice was performed in large municipal "charity" hospitals without generating revenue, no funding agencies for medical research existed, and endowments were inadequate. Little, if any, opportunity for research was available. Medical schools, which were driven by the desire of academic physicians to be medical scholars in a specific field of endeavor, needed to evolve to support research and education in parallel [1,2].

After WW II, the intersection between advances in clinical medicine and physiology, biochemistry, and pharmacology spurred the growth of research in medicine. Young physicians in the post-war period felt tremendous excitement and privilege in becoming clinical investigators mentored by great scientists and clinicians who were also master teachers [3]. Although medical research units of the 1940s were supported almost entirely on private donations and pharmaceutical companies, the burgeoning research institutions of the 1950s and 1960s were beginning to be supported by federal grants and other agencies such as the Howard Hughes Medical Institute, and these institutions began to rival their European counterparts. At these institutions, physicians from all over the world worked together in small units where the patients and laboratories were in close proximity, which made the interaction between clinical medicine and research seamless. The trainees and young faculty were given significant clinical and research responsibilities and had regular, close contact with their mentors. My father, Oscar B. Crofford, was a young researcher in diabetes and metabolism at Vanderbilt University. His recollection of the prevailing charge to young investigators was "go discover something," and young scientists were given extraordinary freedom and support to do just that.

## 12.2 THE DEVELOPMENT OF FEDERAL FUNDING FOR BIOMEDICAL RESEARCH

The expansion of university-based research and training came with the rise of the National Institutes of Health (NIH) from an enterprise with an appropriation of $464,000 in 1938 to more than $1 billion in the late 1960s [4]. The Research Grants Office was created in January 1946 to operate a program of extramural research grants and fellowship awards. The NIH dramatically increased funding for research and postdoctoral training through disease-specific or categorical institutes. The development of these disease-specific institutes and awards led to new divisions within medical schools, including units focused on arthritis and rheumatic diseases. Academic units at the preeminent medical institutions around the country, including the Robert Breck Brigham Hospital, which was the first teaching hospital in the country focused on rheumatic diseases (now Brigham & Women's Hospital at Harvard University); Johns Hopkins University; New York University; Duke University; University of Michigan; University of Texas Southwestern; University of California San Francisco; and University of Washington among others, became a focal point for research and training of scientists in arthritis research through NIH training grants. In the 1960s, according to my father, the success rate of research project grant applications to the NIH was such that almost all feasible and rational applications were funded.

## 12.3   ARTHRITIS RESEARCH AND THE NATIONAL INSTITUTES OF HEALTH

In 1950, the National Institute of Arthritis and Metabolic Diseases was created, and then it evolved to the National Institute of Arthritis, Metabolic, and Digestive Diseases in 1972 [4]. In January 1975, the National Arthritis Act established the National Commission on Arthritis and Related Musculoskeletal Diseases to study the problem of arthritis and develop an arthritis plan. Implementation of the Arthritis plan was given to the National Arthritis Advisory Board and included the development of multipurpose arthritis centers [5,6]. The evolution of the NIH with respect to funding for arthritis research continued with another name change to the National Institute of Arthritis, Diabetes, and Digestive and Kidney Diseases in 1980. The U.S. Department of Health and Human Services conferred bureau status, similar to other major institutes including the National Cancer Institute and National Heart and Lung Institute, in 1982, with a Division of Arthritis and Musculoskeletal and Skin Diseases. In 1986, the National Institute of Arthritis and Musculoskeletal and Skin Diseases (NIAMS) separated from its parent institute. The first director, Dr. Lawrence E. Shulman, served from 1986 to 1994 and presided over growth in the budget from $139 million to $223 million.

In addition to funding extramural research, this was a time of growth for the intramural research program, which had benefited from the amendment to the Selective Service Act in 1950 at the outbreak of the Korean War that allowed entry to the Public Health Service as an alternative to the draft and resulted in the recruitment of a large cadre of extraordinary scientists to the Bethesda campus [7]. The individuals recruited during the so-called "doctor draft" applied to the U.S. Public Health Service Commissioned Corps before being drafted to the armed services and then could be assigned as a clinical associate at the NIH. This resulted in a large number of the best and brightest investigators setting up intramural research programs that flourished for many years. This also benefited NIAMS as a group of outstanding investigators were attracted to the NIH intramural environment. Under the clinical leadership of Dr. John Decker and scientific leadership of Dr. Henry Metzger, the Arthritis and Rheumatism Branch (ARB) of NIAMS was the kind of unit where clinical and laboratory research were carried out in close proximity, trainees were give broad clinical and laboratory roles, and mentors were readily available for scientific discussion. Rheumatologists from across the country and around the world worked in the intramural research program of NIAMS and carried the excitement for science with them to their home institutions. When I was a Clinical Staff Fellow of the ARB between 1989 and 1993, this intramural unit recapitulated the model of the early university-based research units of the 1960s. It was my privilege to work directly with Dr. Shulman to investigate the etiology of the eosinophilia-myalgia syndrome, which clinically mimicked "Shulman's syndrome." Indeed, this was an opportunity to be mentored by a superb scientist and clinician who was also a master teacher.

Dr. Stephen I. Katz has been institute director of NIAMS since 1995 and has presided over growth in the NIAMS budget to over $500 million for the current fiscal year. Despite the growth in the budget, a parallel growth occurred in demand, and the success rate for research project grants, career awards, and training awards has dropped to below 15% for most award mechanisms in the current fiscal year. (http://www.niams.nih.gov/About_Us/Budget/funding_plan_fy2009.asp.) Funding for research in the rheumatic diseases also comes from many other institutes at NIH and from the Department of Veterans Affairs, Centers for Disease Control and Prevention, and other federal agencies that are also experiencing budget shortfalls. However, it is clear that rheumatology researchers must be successful in obtaining federal research funding to sustain an academic career.

## 12.4   THE ARTHRITIS FOUNDATION: A CRITICAL PARTNER IN RESEARCH FUNDING

Foundation funding for medical research has been a critically important adjunct to NIH and other federal funding. In the 1940s, only a few locations in the country existed where physicians and students could gain advanced understanding of diagnosis and treatment of rheumatic diseases. There was widespread pessimism that arthritis could be treated, and less than $11,000 was spent on arthritis research in the country. The members of the American Rheumatism Association, which was the precursor organization to the American College of Rheumatology (ACR), found this situation unacceptable and spearheaded the establishment of the Arthritis and Rheumatism Foundation (http://www.arthritis.org/about-us.php).   Dr. Richard Freyberg of New York identified and recruited a nationally prominent business leader, Floyd Odlum, Chairman of the Board of the Atlas Corporation, to be the first chairman of this new Foundation, and the first meeting was held in 1948. The Foundation began its work by establishing chapters around the country to raise funds. The first campaign was chaired by entertainer Bob Hope and resulted in more than $500,000 to be used to support research and the establishment of specialized arthritis clinics in hospitals.

In 1964, the name was changed to the Arthritis Foundation, and it separated from the American Rheumatism Association. The first long-range plan of the Arthritis Foundation broadened the scope of interest to include all rheumatic diseases with continued goals for fundraising and grant funding to support young and established investigators. The Foundation also developed a robust national peer-review system for evaluating grant applications, and it maintained a program of research funding through some of the individual chapters. Since 1948, the Arthritis Foundation has provided more than $380 million in research grants. Many, if not most, of the established academic rheumatologists and health professionals working today were the recipients of grants such as the Arthritis Investigator award, Biomedical Sciences grants, and Clinical Sciences grants.

Recently, the number of grant mechanisms offered by the Arthritis Foundation have decreased, although the Foundation is still a major contributor to the research effort. A major effort to restructure the Foundation and its chapters to revitalize research funding is underway.

## 12.5 THE ROLE OF INDUSTRY IN MEDICAL RESEARCH

Drastic changes have occurred in the relationship between academicians and the pharmaceutical industry over the years, with rampant pharmaceutical sponsorship in the 1920s leading to the prohibition of patents for faculty in prominent research institutions in the 1930s [8]. The profit motive of industry is still viewed somewhat uneasily by academic medicine and the public, but recent changes to both industry and academia have changed the relationship yet again. Pharmaceutical companies have recruited academic researchers to pursue their own basic research programs in what was previously the purview of traditional university-based scientists [2]. This strategy has been particularly striking in rheumatology where the growth of biologic therapies has led to renewed understanding of disease pathways, as well as to profits that can be reinvested in basic research. A significant number of established and promising young university-based researchers have moved to industry in recent years, which led to the depletion of funded investigators in rheumatology units across the country. Academic scientists and institutions have become more entrepreneurial and thus more comfortable with research as a business [2]. The need for increased funds for research has also led to increased direct institutional support from industry to universities and foundations [2]. A certain wariness remains around conflict of interest in industry-sponsored research concerning the balance between financial benefit for industry and the health benefit to patients. Additional discomfort exists with the notion that gifts from industry may come with real or perceived strings attached. However, it is critical to create and maintain mechanisms that allow industry to contribute to the medical research enterprise in a manner that can be held up to scrutiny and found to be free of conflict of interest.

## 12.6 THE ACR RESEARCH AND EDUCATION FOUNDATION: ENSURING THE FUTURE OF RHEUMATOLOGY

After the separation of the Arthritis Foundation from what is now the ACR, no mechanism was available to provide specific funding for rheumatology and rheumatologists. The goals of other funding agencies differ from those of the ACR; an organization of rheumatologists and rheumatology health professionals must sustain its members. The leadership of the ACR recognized the need to create a foundation specifically to support recruitment, training, and career development of rheumatologists and rheumatology investigators. The ACR Research and Education Foundation (REF) was created to serve this need. At its inception, few staff and little money were available to provide grants to achieve REF goals. A major development in the capacity of the REF to serve its mission came with the development of the Industry Round Table in 2001, whereby pharmaceutical companies provide funds to be used for REF award programs in exchange for recognition of their support, a relationship with the ACR, and benefits that assured exposure for their products at the ACR Annual Scientific Meeting. With this funding as a start, the REF developed a portfolio of research and education awards that observed funding increase from $500,000 in 2000 to more than $5 million in the 2009 budget. This portfolio of "core awards" is designed to promote the specialty to students and residents, provide financial support for subspecialty training in rheumatology, and fund career development for those rheumatologists and health professionals that aspire to a career in research. Furthermore, education awards support senior clinical scholars to develop a new cadre of educators within academic rheumatology units to accomplish ACR and REF goals.

Another major change in the mission of the REF came with the strategic plan of 2005. A measurable reduction had occurred in the proportion of faculty in academic rheumatology units funded by NIH, which accompanied a notable decline in the percentage of successful research project grants from the NIH, reduction in research awards by the Arthritis Foundation, and migration of research to industry. The ACR made the rather bold decision to develop a program to be implemented by the REF that would raise significant funds for disease-targeted research. It was decided that the most appropriate first target was rheumatoid arthritis (RA), which was based on the number of affected individuals, the relatively low federal funding, the feasibility for fundraising, and the potential for significant discovery in basic and clinical science. Although too early to determine the long-term success of the program, the "Within Our Reach" campaign has raised more than $28 million and awarded 45 substantial research grants focused on RA.

Significant challenges are associated with raising funds to support the expanded mission of the REF. The Foundation has now embarked on a goal to set aside an endowment to secure our ability to fund recruitment, training, and career development over the long term. This will certainly require the REF to increase the donor base and to develop a planned giving program only recently implemented. How disease-targeted research will evolve remains unclear, but the need for the ACR and REF to support research in the rheumatic diseases is unlikely to diminish in the foreseeable future.

## 12.7  CONCLUSIONS

The evolution from my grandfather's experience, to the focused and integrated clinical research units where my father trained, to the hugely complex and often fragmented enterprise that we recognize today will surely continue [2]. Although there are many threats to the survival of the academic physicians and research units that advance basic and clinical research in the rheumatic diseases, the enormous satisfaction of pursuing basic and applied research in academia remains. The challenge for academic rheumatology is to stay focused on the great rewards of the work and the academic environment. There are concerning trends that include physicians being evaluated to a significant extent by whether they "cover their salary" with clinical revenue or research funding. With the difficulties in obtaining the funding necessary to complete the complex and expensive studies that use new technology, many academic physicians are pressed to generate clinical revenue and have reduced time spent in mentoring. The time demands required to generate support leaves precious little time to think creatively about research and to incorporate what we learn from our patients into our thinking. The REF will continue to work toward an award program that complements other funding programs to address our challenges while the ACR advocates for stable rheumatic disease research funding at NIH and other federal agencies.

A return to past models where clinical medicine, education, and research take place simultaneously and in an integrated fashion seems almost unattainable, but it is a goal worthy of attention. Certainly, room for hope exists with some of the changes outlined by the NIH roadmap. Perhaps recognizing deficiencies in academic medicine of today, initiatives including the Clinical and Translational Science Award program at the NIH seek to reestablish the link between the practice of medicine, research, and education that will promote translation of discovery to advance the prevention and treatment of patients with arthritis and rheumatic diseases.

## REFERENCES

1. Ludmerer KM. Learning to Heal. New York: Basic Books, Inc; 1985.
2. Feinstein AR. Scholars, investigators, and entrepreneurs. The metamorphosis of American medicine. Perspect Biol Med 2003;46:234–253.
3. Swazey JP, Fox RC. Remembering the "golden years" of patient-oriented clinical research: A collective conversation. Perspect Biol Med 2004;47:487–504.
4. National Institute of Health NIH Almanac 2008–2009. p. 400–403.
5. Engelman EP. The national arthritis plan: An overview. Arthritis Rheum 1977;20:1–6.
6. Singsen BH, Winfield JB, Brandt KD, Rothfield NF, Hausman SJ. Multipurpose arthritis centers. A ten-year progress report. Arthritis Rheum 1988;31:1574–1583.
7. Park BS. The development of the intramural research program at the National Institutes of Health after World War II. Perspect Biol Med 2003;46:383–402.
8. Rasmussen N. The drug industry and clinical research in interwar America: Three types of physician collaborator. Bull Hist Med 2005;79:50–80.

Chapter *13*

# Changes in Practice Since 1975

**Neal S. Birnbaum**

*Pacific Rheumatology Association, San Francisco, CA*

I joined the American College of Rheumatology (ACR) in 1975 as a first-year fellow under Dr. Gerald Rodnan at the University of Pittsburgh. Moving to San Francisco to begin practice 2 years later, it seemed natural to continue my membership. Although I never think of myself as a "mature" practitioner, I have been an ACR member for nearly half of the organization's 75-year history.

In thinking about changes in practice over the past three plus decades, it is tempting to immediately talk about the dramatic advances in therapeutics for inflammatory arthritis brought about by the advent of biologics in the late 1990s. Prior to that time, rheumatology had really been stuck in the doldrums for nearly my entire practice life. I started to use methotrexate around 1980 and did not have anything else new until leflunomide and etanercept nearly two decades later. Lupus treatment remains controversial, particularly for life-threatening organ involvement, and scleroderma is nearly as frustrating to manage today as when I was the scleroderma fellow with Dr. Rodnan and Dr. Thomas Medsger. Allopurinol had been in use prior to my entering the field of rheumatology and only very recently have additional agents been developed for gout, which is the most historic of the rheumatic disorders.

I have spent my entire career in small-group private practice. Thinking back to my first office in 1977, I realized that much of the electronic connectivity that we take for granted today did not exist at that time. Copying machines were rudimentary, using

*The ACR at 75: A Diamond Jubilee*
Copyright © 2009 by John Wiley & Sons, Inc.

coated paper that quickly faded and turned yellow. Obtaining laboratory or radiology reports from the local hospital required waiting for days or having a staff person laboriously hand copy the results given over the phone. Eventually, facsimile reports became routine and are now being quickly supplanted by computerized access. It is not that long ago that physicians on call knew the location of every pay telephone and always had a pocket full of quarters, or was it dimes? I remember thinking that a cell phone really was a luxury rather than a necessity! I may be one of the few who still feels that way about a Blackberry.

The business of medicine has changed dramatically over the years. In my first years of practice, patients actually received a bill and were expected to pay their doctor for the services received. What they were reimbursed from their insurance company was a matter left to the patient and the carrier. In the 1980s, traditional private health insurance began to give way to various preferred provider organization (PPO) and health maintenance organization (HMO) products. Initial contracts between insurance carriers and physicians usually paid at or near "usual and customary fees" as long as the charges were not grossly out of line. However, that situation changed as the merger of insurers into megacarriers gave them bargaining clout that physicians have rarely been able to challenge successfully. Medicare, once one of the worst payers, is now considered better than many private insurers in certain parts of the country.

Many internists, particularly rheumatologists, made much of their income from providing in-office ancillary services. Undercutting of fees by large commercial laboratories has driven many physician office laboratories out of business. My patients loved the convenience of not having to wait in a long line to have their blood drawn at the much more expensive hospital-owned laboratory down the hall. However, when I shut down our in-office lab 10 years ago, the practice was losing $3,000 each month providing this service. Although I have never provided bone density testing in our office, I know that marked reduction in Medicare reimbursement has recently forced many rheumatologists to give up their dual-energy x-ray absorptiometry (DEXA) machines. These trends make it so important for the ACR to continue its long fight for improved reimbursement for evaluation and management services. It has been shown time and again that everything but our cognitive skills can be taken away by unreasonable reimbursement schemes. I often remind colleagues that I now do infusions in the room that used to be the office laboratory. I suspect that newer self-injected biologics and oral small-molecule therapies will eventually make in-office infusion obsolete.

Nothing has changed the practice of medicine as rapidly and dramatically as the advent of computers. What started out as a toy for "geeks" who were likely engineering majors before they went to medical school soon became an indispensable part of every practice. The first rudimentary computer in my office was used only by the billing clerk. It was not until several years later that a computer arrived on my desk. Before long, "Do you have e-mail?" was replaced by "What's your e-mail address?" UpToDate and Google searches have largely replaced the use of textbooks and doing research at the hospital library. A year ago, I emptied out the large file cabinet that housed thousands of paper journal articles that I had religiously clipped and filed dating back to medical school at Ohio State. I was nervous that I would miss having those "classic" studies at my fingertips for both teaching and patient care. So far, I have not had a single instance where I could not manage perfectly well with the literature rapidly available to me on the Internet. Although I cannot imagine living without e-mail connectivity during my term as ACR president in 2006–2007, I have been reluctant to communicate with patients in that way. I find it invaluable to hear a patient's voice and interact in real time. In addition, I can talk far faster than I can type!

Of course, it is not just physicians who have access to computers. I used to be the primary source for educating my patients, keeping a large supply of Arthritis Foundation pamphlets and other printed materials on hand. Now, patients often have done their own computerized literature searches before coming to the office. They frequently have made their own diagnoses and researched the treatment options. Now my job includes interpreting this information as to its accuracy and applicability to that individual.

Like many practices, our office is in the midst of converting to an electronic health record (EHR). By the time this article is published, we will hopefully be well on our way to a paperless office with connectivity to hundreds of other physicians in our large independent practice association (IPA). Already I can access my appointment schedule from home or even on vacation as well as view diagnostic studies and inpatient records from several hospitals and commercial laboratories. It has been a bit of a struggle for people like me who have always done well with a paper chart. Younger physicians who grew up playing Pac-Man seem to have an easier time than those of us from the pinball generation! I have yet to see an EHR that saves the physician a great deal of time, and I worry about the temporary loss of productivity that even strong technology advocates admit accompanies the conversion to an electronic chart.

Despite all that has changed in the practice of rheumatology over the past 34 years, I am actually amazed at how much has stayed the same. Entering the consultation or exam room really hasn't changed much at all. As I wrote in a 2007 presidential column in *The Rheumatologist*, I still enjoy being a rheumatologist and have no regrets about my chosen specialty. Both patients and fellow physicians seem to respect the rheumatologist's role as a medical detective and expert diagnostician. A detailed history and physical examination remain more likely to provide a proper diagnosis than a battery of ancillary studies. Promising a young man with gout that he will soon be free of painful attacks is just as much fun as it was as a fellow. Reassuring an older woman that her months of disabling nighttime pain and morning stiffness caused by polymyalgia rheumatica will be gone within a few hours of starting low-dose prednisone is as gratifying now as when I first entered practice. Winning the confidence of an anxious, new mother referred for lupus and reassuring her that her antinuclear antibody (ANA) is a false positive is still as rewarding as it was at the beginning of my career. Perhaps it is even a bit easier now that I have the gray hair of a seasoned practitioner. Even if my retirement plan makes a rapid recovery, I suspect that I will be going to the office and enjoying the practice of rheumatology for years to come.

# Chapter *14*

# *Multidisciplinary Rheumatology*

**Marian A. Minor**

*University of Missouri, Physical Therapy, Columbia, MO*

In 1965, as I started my career as a physical therapist, my first patient was a woman with rheumatoid arthritis, Functional Class IV. She had been treated with high-dose corticosteroids for over 15 years and was admitted to the rehabilitation unit for 2 weeks every summer. The orders were for mat exercises (passive and active-assisted range of motion) in the morning and ambulation in the parallel bars in the afternoon. As a student, I had received one lecture on rheumatoid arthritis (RA) and attended grand rounds about corticosteroids. I remembered that RA was probably some kind of autoimmune disease and that long-term corticosteroids had serious consequences. I understood a bit about my patient's osteoporosis, fragile skin, and muscle atrophy but not much more than that.

My patient's experiences had taught her that she always was assigned to the most junior therapists and that her pain increased with our treatment attempts. She had learned how to keep us engaged in conversation to stave off therapy and how to maintain some control over her life by dire warnings of imminent bowel and bladder needs. I learned a lot from her—a proud, farm woman who lived with a consuming disease and had received treatment that produced even more disability. She gave me much more than I gave to her.

*The ACR at 75: A Diamond Jubilee*
Copyright © 2009 by John Wiley & Sons, Inc.

When I was observing my first patient, many medical schools did not have formal rheumatology programs, health professional curricula contained little training in rheumatic disease, and multidisciplinary team care was not the norm. It was not until the 1970s that publications began to appear to describe a team approach for arthritis and events unfolded to support multidisciplinary care and research.

## 14.1   MULTIDISCIPLINARY CARE

Originally, multidisciplinary care was hospital-based team care. Early studies of effectiveness examined outcomes from inpatient rheumatic disease units and from multidisciplinary inputs at outpatient follow-ups. Most evidence to support forma-lized multidisciplinary care has come from studies in rheumatoid arthritis [1]. Advances in treatment and changes in health-care delivery have reduced inpatient stays, and multidisciplinary care is evolving to serve in outpatient and community settings. Models of care vary for types of disease and the delivery system.

In 2008, MacKay et al. [2] identified five models of multidisciplinary care in Canada, Europe, Scandinavia, and Australia. Models ranged from conventional clinical and hospital-based care, to expanded clinical roles for nurses and physical therapists, to rural consultation and telemedicine. Whatever the context, effective multidisciplinary care is founded on knowledgeable health care providers with well-defined roles; effective methods of communication; a patient-centered, coordinated approach to management across the continuum; and education to teach self-management skills. Recognition of the need for a multidisciplinary and coordinated approach to manage-ment of rheumatic disease entered public policy in the United States in 1977.

## 14.2   NIH MULTIPURPOSE ARTHRITIS CENTERS

The U.S. National Arthritis Act of 1975 grew out of congressional hearings and established a National Commission on Arthritis and Musculoskeletal Disease that presented the first National Arthritis Plan in 1977. Among other recommendations, the plan called for funding arthritis centers throughout the country. The ensuing call for proposals for Multipurpose Arthritis Center (MAC) applications described a MAC as a:

> . . . . Group of formally cooperating health personnel . . . brought together to demonstrate and foster the prompt and effective application of available knowledge and the devel-opment of urgently needed new knowledge. . . . must include activities in three major fields: education, research and community-related activities. . . . Shall conduct: basic and clinical research related to the causes, diagnosis, early detection, prevention, control and treatment of arthritis and related complications; training programs for physicians and other health and allied professionals; information and continuing education for physicians and other allied health professionals, and program for dissemination of information to the general public [3].

The vision and call for integrated, multidisciplinary knowledge and care was clear. The National Institutes of Health (NIH) funded the first MACs in 1977. An important task of these early MACs was to promote a scholarly (research) component of education and community-related efforts and training for more pediatric rheumatologists, orthopedists, physiatrists, and allied health professionals skilled in arthritis care and research [4].

The impact of MACs on the number and diversity of health professionals committed to rheumatology care and research was remarkable. Membership of the American Rheumatism Association (ARA) and the Arthritis Health Professions Association (AHPA) doubled in the first 10 years of MAC funding. The number of scientific presentation at ARA and AHPA annual meetings rose from 342 in 1976–1978 to 649 in 1987 (clinical/laboratory research rose from 78 to 84 sessions and education/health services research (HSR)/behavioral research rose from 14 to 61 sessions). MAC personnel comprised about 20% of ARA presentations and about 38% of AHPA presentations [4]. MACs required and supported research and scholarly capacity building in a variety of health professions—medicine, basic science, nursing, occupational therapy, physical therapy, psychology, social work, and health education, to name but a few.

In 1988 the ARA moved to establish an autonomous organization, the American College of Rheumatology (ACR). In 1994, the AHPA joined the ACR as a Division, the Association of Rheumatology Health Professionals (ARHP).

## 14.3 ACR/ARHP: A MULTIDISCIPLINARY PROFESSIONAL ORGANIZATION

When ARHP joined ACR, collaborative administrative infrastructure and joint annual scientific meetings were established. The combined annual scientific meetings have provided the recurring venue for scholarly dialog and professional relationships among many disciplines. The merger set the stage for widespread collegial and multidisciplinary perspectives to emerge in rheumatology care and research.

In 2001, ACR/ARHP received a National Institute of Arthritis and Musculoskeletal and Skin Diseases (NIAMS) conference grant. The International Conference on Health Promotion and Disability Prevention for Individuals and Populations with Rheumatic Disease: The Evidence for Exercise and Physical Activity was held in March 2002. Presenters represented the fields of rheumatology, physical therapy, nursing, biomechanics, psychology, epidemiology, public health, health services research, and exercise physiology. Proceedings were disseminated as papers and work group recommendations in a series in *Arthritis Care and Research (AC&R)* in 2003 (49:1–3) and as a monograph supported by the Arthritis Program, National Center for Chronic Disease Prevention and Health Promotion, Centers for Disease Control and Prevention.

In 2003 and 2007, ACR/ARHP issued a position statement on multidisciplinary care calling for "timely and affordable access to multidisciplinary care and rehabilitation services for patients with rheumatic and musculoskeletal diseases."

ARHP developed and launched the Nurse Practitioner and Physician Assistant Postgraduate Rheumatology Training Program in 2008. This self-study provides training and certification in rheumatologic care for these professions, which are a growing component of membership and increasingly active as care providers.

The ACR Rehabilitative Rheumatology Section has proposed a name change to reflect its longstanding interdisciplinary membership. When approved, the section will become the Section on Interdisciplinary Arthritis Management (IAM) in 2009.

The ACR Research and Education Foundation offers awards for ACR and ARHP members including predoctoral and postdoctoral awards and grants for new and established clinical investigators.

## 14.4   MULTIDISCIPLINARY PUBLICATIONS

*AC&R* (first published in 1988, with editor, Donna Hawley, RN, PhD) became an ACR/ARHP publication. The mission of the journal was evaluated and revised in 1999, and Gene Hunder, MD, became editor in 2000. Patti Katz, PhD, and Ed Yelin, PhD, were selected as coeditors in 2004. In response to the rapidly growing number and quality of submissions, *AC&R* became a monthly publication in 2008. The purpose of *AC&R* is multidisciplinary. The journal publishes papers on evidence-based practice studies, clinical problems, practice guidelines, health care economics, health care policy, educational, social, and public health issues, and future trends in rheumatology practice. A major multidisciplinary contribution by *AC&R* was publication of the supplement, Patient Outcomes in Rheumatology in 2003.

*Clinical Care in the Rheumatic Diseases*, originally conceived as a companion publication to the *Primer on Rheumatic Diseases*, was first published in 1996 with subsequent editions in 2001 and 2006. In the most recent edition, over 80 contributing authors addressed a wide range of topics related to clinical care of patients with a range of rheumatic diseases [5].

Practice guidelines for RA and osteoarthritis (OA) clearly support both pharmacologic and nonpharmacologic care with multiple interventions requiring knowledgeable practitioners in several disciplines [6,7].

## 14.5   IN CONCLUSION

In the United States, the 1977 National Arthritis Act and the NIH MAC program initiated work that produced a critical mass of researchers and clinicians from a range of disciplines relevant to rheumatology. The ACR/ARHP, which is an international, multidisciplinary professional organization centered on rheumatic disease, provides ongoing opportunities for clinicians and scientists from around the world to discover and share new knowledge as well as to learn, teach, and implement better ways to care for people with arthritis. The MAC programs infused energy and personnel into multidisciplinary rheumatology. ACR/ARHP supports the ongoing evolution of this perspective. It has been 44 years since I saw my first patient with arthritis. In years, it does not seem that long ago; in the progress in rheumatology, it is a world—a lifetime—of difference for the better.

## REFERENCES

1. Vliet Vlieland TP. Multidisciplinary team care and outcomes in rheumatoid arthritis. Curr Opin Rheumatol 2004;16:153–156.
2. MacKay C, Veinot P, Badley EM. Characteristics of evolving models of care for arthritis: A key informant study. BMC Health Serv Res 2008;8:147.
3. National Institutes of Health. NIH Guide for grants and contracts. USDHEW. 1977;6:2–3.
4. Singsen BH, Winfield JB, Brandt KD, Rothfield NF, Hausman SJ. Multipurpose arthritis centers, a ten-year progress report. Arthritis Rheum 1988;31:1574–1583.
5. Bartlett SJ (ed). Clinical Care in the Rheumatic Diseases (3rd ed.). Atlanta, GA: Association of Rheumatology Health Professionals; 2006.
6. American College of Rheumatology. Practice Guidelines. Available: http://www.rheumatology.org/publications/guidelines/index.asp?aud=mem.
7. Jordan KM, Arden NK, Doherty M, et al. EULAR Recommendations 2003: an evidence-based approach to the management of knee osteoarthritis: Report of a Task force of the Standing Committee for International Clinical Studies including therapeutic Trials (ESCISIT). Ann Rheum Dis 2003;62:1145–1155.

# Chapter 15

# Developments in Surgery for Rheumatic and Musculoskeletal Disorders

**Jeffrey N. Katz**

*Brigham and Women's Hospital, Rheumatology, Boston, MA*

The past 75 years have witnessed remarkable advances in orthopedic surgery for musculoskeletal and rheumatic diseases. This chapter attempts to capture the highlights, starting with one of the most extraordinary advances in modern medicine: total joint replacement surgery (TJR) for advanced arthritis.

## 15.1 TOTAL JOINT REPLACEMENT SURGERY

In the 1940s and 1950s, advanced joint destruction from osteoarthritis, rheumatoid arthritis, and other joint diseases accounted for substantial wheelchair dependence, nursing home use, and premature loss of productivity. In one of the most extraordinary advances in 20th-century medicine, Sir John Charnley, working in Wrightington, England, introduced total hip replacement in the 1960s. By the late 1970s, hip replacement had advanced from pioneering science to routine care and was performed throughout the United States and Europe. Hip replacement provided unprecedented

*The ACR at 75: A Diamond Jubilee*
Copyright © 2009 by John Wiley & Sons, Inc.

relief of pain and gain in function for patients who previously had to drop out of productive life.

Similar advances in total knee replacement followed, and by the 1980s, total knee replacement was also performed throughout the developed world. The early history of total hip and total knee replacement was characterized by innovations in device design, materials engineering, and hospital care to address the challenges of superficial and deep joint infection, dislocation, early loosening, and later component failure. By the turn of the 21st century, infection and mortality rates in the first 90 days after hip and knee replacements were less than 1% [1,2]. The typical hip and knee replacement can now be expected to last more than 20 years [3,4].

These advances catalyzed a paradigm shift in the use of total joint replacement surgery. Initially reserved for patients with far advanced functional decline caused by painful, end-stage arthritis, joint replacement surgery is now offered to patients at much higher levels of function so that they can continue to perform activities essential for maintaining role functions at work and home. In fact, patients who undergo surgery at an earlier point in the trajectory of functional decline have better functional outcomes than patients operated on at a worse level of function [5]. Joint replacement is offered increasingly to younger, active patients with early advanced arthritis, such as the 48 year old with hip osteoarthritis caused by congenital dysplasia. These active patients present technical challenges. They wear their prostheses faster and have longer projected life expectancy. Current innovation focuses on developing biomaterials and approaches, such as ceramic and metal bearing surfaces and hip resurfacing, which best serve these young active patients. Whether these innovations will overcome the technical challenge of early failure in young active TJR recipients awaits careful follow-up studies. Indications are also expanding to include older patients, as perioperative management has reduced the risk of medical complications.

It has been projected that total knee replacements, currently done on 500,000 persons per year in the United States, will be offered to as many as 3.5 million persons per year by the year 2030 [6]. These extraordinary projections suggest that total joint replacement, which was initially a "specialty item" concentrated in research centers, will become a medical commodity. How the health care system and various providers deal with this transition from specialty to commodity care will define financial winners and losers. Whether our patients will be winners depends on the thoughtfulness of these transitions and the sorts of incentives and programs offered by the federal government and other major insurers.

## 15.2    IMAGING AND THE SURGICAL IMPERATIVE: YOU CANNOT FIX WHAT YOU CANNOT SEE

Another extraordinary set of technological advances in the last 75 years relate to imaging and minimally invasive surgery. Magnetic resonance imaging (MRI), which was developed in the 1970s, and introduced into widespread clinical use by the 1990s, has provided unprecedented, detailed views of numerous musculoskeletal structures including the spine, knee, shoulder, and others. Spine imaging essentially created a new disorder called lumbar spinal stenosis. Although well described in the early part of the 20th century, spinal stenosis could only be detected with myelography, which is an invasive technique. Thus, the diagnosis was made infrequently. The introduction of noninvasive cross-sectional imaging, first with computed tomography and then with MRI, facilitated structural diagnosis. Spinal stenosis is now the leading indication for spine surgery in the elderly. Decompression for stenosis is performed on over 250,000 patients annually in the United States.

The capacity to image the knee, shoulder, hip, wrist, elbow, and ankle, among other structures, has also permitted the noninvasive diagnosis of meniscal tears, cruciate ligament injuries, labral tears in the hip, labral and rotator cuff tears in the shoulder, ligamentous lesions of the wrist, and other disorders. Each of these problems can be addressed with arthroscopic surgery. The expanding capacity of the orthopedic workforce in operating rooms across the country and attractive financial remuneration for performing these procedures have led to an increase in the use of arthroscopy for knee, hip, and shoulder disorders. Knee arthroscopy, for example, is performed on over one million persons in the United States annually. Evidence to support the efficacy of most arthroscopic procedures is thin. Two high-quality trials reported in the last decade documented that arthroscopic lavage and debridement for knee osteoarthritis offer no advantages over sham surgery or a nonoperative regimen [7,8]. Arthroscopic rotator cuff repair and arthroscopic partial meniscal resection have not been addressed in rigorous, large, randomized controlled trials reported to date.

## 15.3 TREATING THE PATIENT AND NOT THE SCAN...

The ready availability of cross-sectional imaging and noninvasive surgery has proved to be a two-edged sword. What is a "normal" MRI in an adult? Over 20% of *asymptomatic* adults have rotator cuff tears, meniscal tears, lumbar disc protrusions, lumbar spinal stenosis, cervical stenosis, or combinations of these lesions [9–12]. Thus, the presence of pain coupled with a surgically amenable lesion on imaging does not necessarily create an indication for surgery. If the anatomic lesion (e.g., a meniscal tear) occurs in more than one fifth of asymptomatic individuals, it can certainly occur in symptomatic individuals and yet not be responsible for the symptoms and attendant disability. Ironically, as diagnostic technology advances, we have become increasingly dependent on the history and physical examination to put structural findings into a clinical context.

## 15.4 THE EPIDEMIC OF ANTERIOR CRUCIATE LIGAMENT TEARS

The frequencies of anterior cruciate ligament injuries and surgical repairs have increased rapidly in the last 30 years, particularly in women. Although the increased recognition and treatment of these lesions occurred in part from the availability of MRI and arthroscopic surgery, the epidemic also stemmed from one of the most progressive pieces of U.S. legislation of the last century. Title IX of the Federal Education Amendments of 1972 mandated equal funding of women's and men's sports at the collegiate and high-school levels. Participation by high-school girls in interscholastic sports increased 10-fold since the passage of Title IX. The same period witnessed a dramatic increase in anterior cruciate ligament tears in young women [13].

The reasons these tears have occurred so much more frequently in females than in males are not entirely clear but seem to include gender differences in anatomy, hormonal milieu, and in athletic technique, such as pivoting, jumping, and landing. Preventive efforts to address these risk factors have been proposed but are not supported with rigorous trials at this point. These injuries have led to a rapid increase in the use of surgery to repair anterior cruciate ligaments. This area of technological advance has been active with respect to surgical approach, graft material, post-operative rehabilitation, and surgical indications. The growing evidence that joint instability leads to premature osteoarthritis has heightened the need for accurate diagnosis and early intervention of cruciate ligament tears.

## 15.5 INFLAMMATORY ARTHRITIS: SURGERY ON THE WANE

Medical advances have reduced the need for some surgical approaches. Remarkable advances in the management of inflammatory arthritis with disease modifying agents, particularly tumor necrosis factor (TNF) inhibitors, have changed the role of surgery for these conditions. Early evidence is emerging that total joint replacement, fusion, and other procedures that address the structural complications of inflammatory arthritis are used less frequently in patients with inflammatory arthritis now than decades ago because of successes in controlling inflammation with early aggressive biologic therapy [14,15].

## 15.6 THE FUTURE

What advances will occur in the next 75 years? The disciplinary boundaries between medical and surgical specialties will become increasingly blurred. Orthopedic surgeons offer patients the opportunity to apply biologic therapies locally. We have examples already including autologous chondrocyte implantation for knee cartilage defect [16]. Trials are under way using surgical approaches to gene therapy for inflammatory arthritis and osteoarthritis. Stem-cell research is likely to produce additional approaches to tissue engineering that will be delivered to patients through collaborative teams of surgeons, rheumatologists, imaging specialists, and engineers. It is easy to envision the field of musculoskeletal medicine evolving similarly to vascular medicine, in which collaborative teams representing surgical medical imaging, pharmacy, and rehabilitative disciplines work together to address the complex needs of patients with musculoskeletal disorders.

# REFERENCES

1. Mahomed NN, Barrett J, Katz JN, et al. Epidemiology of total knee replacement in the United States Medicare population. J Bone Joint Surg Am 2005;87:1222–1228.
2. Mahomed NN, Barrett JA, Katz JN, et al. Rates and outcomes of primary and revision total hip replacement in the United States medicare population. J Bone Joint Surg Am 2003;85-A:27–32.
3. Malchau H, Garellick G, Eisler T, et al. Presidential guest address: The Swedish Hip Registry: increasing the sensitivity by patient outcome data. Clin Orthop Relat Res 2005;441:19–29.
4. Gioe TJ, Sinner P, Mehle S, Ma W, Killeen KK. Excellent survival of all-polyethylene tibial components in a community joint registry. Clin Orthop Relat Res 2007;464:88–92.
5. Fortin PR, Penrod JR, Clarke AE, et al. Timing of total joint replacement affects clinical outcomes among patients with osteoarthritis of the hip or knee. Arthritis Rheum 2002;46:3327–3330.
6. Kurtz S, Ong K, Lau E, et al. Projections of primary and revision hip and knee arthroplasty in the United States from 2005 to 2030. J Bone Joint Surg Am 2007;89:780–785.
7. Kirkley A, Birmingham TB, Litchfield RB, et al. A randomized trial of arthroscopic surgery for osteoarthritis of the knee. N Engl J Med 2008;359:1097–1107.
8. Moseley JB, O'Malley K, Petersen NJ, et al. A controlled trial of arthroscopic surgery for osteoarthritis of the knee. N Engl J Med 2002;347:81–88.
9. Boden SD, McCowin PR, Davis DO, et al. Abnormal magnetic-resonance scans of the cervical spine in asymptomatic subjects. A prospective investigation. J Bone Joint Surg Am 1990;72:1178–1184.
10. Jensen MC, Brant-Zawadzki MN, Obuchowski N, et al. Magnetic resonance imaging of the lumbar spine in people without back pain. N Engl J Med 1994;331:69–73.
11. Englund M, Guermazi A, Gale D, et al. Incidental meniscal findings on knee MRI in middle-aged and elderly persons. N Engl J Med 2008;359:1108 1115.
12. Reilly P, Macleod I, Macfarlane R, et al. Dead men and radiologists don't lie: A review of cadaveric and radiological studies of rotator cuff tear prevalence. Ann R Coll Surg Engl 2006;88:116–121.
13. Hewett TE, Myer GD, Ford KR, et al. Dynamic neuromuscular analysis training for preventing anterior cruciate ligament injury in female athletes. Instr Course Lect 2007;56:397–406.
14. Weiss RJ, Ehlin A, Montgomery SM, et al. Decrease of RA-related orthopaedic surgery of the upper limbs between 1998 and 2004: Data from 54,579 Swedish RA inpatients. Rheumatology (Oxford) 2008;47:491–494.
15. da Silva E, Doran MF, Crowson CS, et al. Declining use of orthopedic surgery in patients with rheumatoid arthritis? Results of a long-term, population-based assessment. Arthritis Rheum 2003;49:216–220.
16. Brun P, Dickinson SC, Zavan B, et al. Characteristics of repair tissue in second-look and third-look biopsies from patients treated with engineered cartilage: Relationship to symptomatology and time after implantation. Arthritis Res Ther 2008;10:R132.

# Chapter 16

# The More Things Change: Health Services Research in the Rheumatic Diseases

**Edward H. Yelin**

*Arthritis Research Group, University of California, San Francisco, CA*

Health services research has been defined most broadly as ". . . the multidisciplinary field of scientific investigation that studies how social factors, financing systems, organizational structures and processes, health technologies, and personal behaviors affect access to health care, the quality and cost of health care, and ultimately our health and well-being. Its research domains are individuals, families, organizations, institutions, communities, and populations" [1].

I have been lucky to sustain a career in this kind of research since the mid-1970s when it was first recognized as a field and adopted by the rheumatology community to address concerns about persons with rheumatic diseases and their health care. Since that time, the scope of inquiry for health services research in rheumatology has expanded from its initial focus on access to and cost of care and measurement of outcomes to encompass the impact of the ways that care is organized on outcomes, the effect of community on the expression of disease, and the interaction between the genetic makeup of the individual and the nature of the environment on the onset and progress of specific rheumatic conditions.

Concurrently, the sophistication of the methods has increased and makes our early efforts seem pedestrian, or even suspect. The kinds of information now available are astounding and include administrative and clinical data that capture the universe of the beneficiaries of the Medicare program as well as of private health plans, or, better yet, all residents of Canadian provinces or health districts in the United Kingdom.

Finally, the nature of the research has shifted from *descriptive* studies to *analytic* ones with clear-cut implications for changes in clinical treatment and public policy.

If one were to ask notable health services researchers in rheumatology to list signature developments in our field, they would no doubt cite different papers. My own list stems from the observation that until the last decade or so, effective treatments were limited. In that situation, persons with rheumatic diseases had to grab onto whatever could be shown to yield improved outcomes, even if effects were small. Thus, I would include as important the following developments in the field: studies establishing that rheumatologists achieved better outcomes for rheumatoid arthritis (RA) and, perhaps, gout conditions [2]; studies establishing that until recently, persons with discrete rheumatic diseases cared for in managed care received similar kinds and amounts of care and experienced similar outcomes as those in fee-for-service settings [3,4] (that situation may be changing based on the high cost of contemporary treatments and the erosion of health insurance coverage) [5,6]; studies showing the benefit of receiving care from a high-volume provider or institution [7–10]; and studies documenting both the existence of racial and gender disparities in care [11–14]; and the reasons for such disparities [15–19].

Beyond studies of the health care system, however, a defining characteristic of much of the best health services research in the rheumatic diseases is its objective to overcome the perception that rheumatic diseases are not as impactful as other major conditions, such as cancer and heart disease, because they are not considered major causes of mortality.

As a consequence, seminal work has been conducted to develop outcome indices that highlight the profound impact of the rheumatic diseases on functioning and quality of life. This work started with the publication in the same issue of *Arthritis and Rheumatism* in 1980 of what are two of the most frequently used measures in rheumatology, the Health Assessment Questionnaire (HAQ) and Arthritis Impact Measurement Scales (AIMS) [20,21]. Progress in treatment of rheumatic conditions may be marked by the fact that the measures have had to be refined to account for smaller gradations in benefit at the highest levels of functioning [22]. Indeed, persons with rheumatic diseases may no longer be satisfied with being able to do *basic* activities of daily living such as ambulation and toileting but, instead, expect treatments that can help them retain more integrative activities such as work, social relationships, and leisure time pursuits, which are together called "valued life activities" [23]. Another manifestation of the effort to convey the importance of the rheumatic diseases has been studies of their economic impacts. The studies have been of two kinds: those about specific discrete rheumatic conditions, particularly rheumatoid arthritis, and those of the entire rubric. The first-generation studies on the costs of rheumatoid arthritis showed that the largest share of total costs was associated with the cessation or reduction of employment [24]. Within the health care component, the largest share of costs was from hospitalizations for total joint replacement, even though fewer than 1 in 10 persons with RA incurred these costs in any 1 year. The development of biological-response-modifying agents has dramatically altered the picture, with some U.S. series indicating that upward of 30% of persons with RA were receiving a biologic, with the costs perhaps eclipsing those due to work loss [5,25,26]. In the studies of all forms of rheumatic diseases in the nation as a whole, researchers have observed that the economic impact of this group of conditions has grown substantially over the last four decades. This impact is related to the aging of the population; lessened mortality from other causes, which has the paradoxical effect of extending the period of disability; and the growing expense of treatment [27–30].

A major contribution to the effort to document the impact of the rheumatic diseases was completed by the sociologist Dr. Lois Verbrugge. Dr. Verbrugge first showed that men and women tend to get different chronic diseases, with men predominating in fatal ones, whereas women have higher rates of nonfatal ones, which include arthritis and neurological impairment [31]. She then went on to compare the impact of seven leading chronic diseases and showed that arthritis is the top-ranked cause of disability and ambulatory care encounters, but it is not among the leading causes of hospital care or of mortality. She concluded with the observation that nonfatal conditions do not receive the attention of policy makers in proportion to their impact [32].

But perhaps the longest running theme in health services research in the rheumatic diseases, and one shared by those studying persons with other conditions (or with none for that matter), is the role that health insurance or its lack plays in health care access and use. This is the subject, directly, of my first peer-reviewed article [33] and indirectly of about half published subsequently, and more importantly is the subject of intense political debate in regular cycles since the Great Depression [34]. It is again a subject of concern, study, and speculation. No consistent data sources are available to track our progress in providing adequate health care coverage for persons with arthritis over the decades. However, in an analysis of the Medical Expenditures Panel Survey (MEPS), fielded over the last decade, we can measure our progress—or, sadly, the lack of it—over this period. Between 1996 and 2005, the last year for which MEPS data are available, the proportion of all persons with arthritis and related conditions without health insurance has hovered between 6% and 7%, although among the poor with arthritis, the proportion without health insurance has increased by about a quarter. However, there has been an erosion of the proportion with private insurance (including those with Medicare plus a Medi-gap policy), from 75% in the first year to 68% in the last year. In contrast, the proportion of persons with coverage *only* from public sector programs, principally Medicare and Medicaid, has increased *dramatically*, from 19% to 25%, or by just under a third in relative terms.

However, as outlined by Lurie and colleagues using MEPS data for the years 1998 through 2004 [35] and in an analysis for this chapter for the period from 1996 through 2005, out-of-pocket expenditures among persons with arthritis, regardless of insurance status, have soared. Between 1996 and 2005, the median out-of-pocket expenditures among all persons with arthritis doubled in constant dollars, from $384 to $762. Among such persons who lack insurance, however, these expenditures more than tripled, albeit from a lower initial base.

Thus, three decades after the first health services research papers in the rheumatic diseases were published, health care coverage for persons with these conditions is no more common (and, among those who are poor, substantially less common), but the out-of-pocket burden of care is much higher, dramatically so among those without insurance. Proposed solutions to this dilemma differ across the political spectrum, just as they have for much of the post-war period. The paradox is that we know much more about the burdens faced by those with rheumatic diseases and their origin, but we seem no closer in this nation to redressing those burdens or sharing them more equitably.

## REFERENCES

1. AcademyHealth. What is Health Services Research. 2000. Available: http://www.academyhealth.org/hsrproj/definitionofhsr.htm.
2. Solomon D, Bates D, Panush R, et al. Costs, outcomes, and patient satisfaction by provider type for patients with rheumatic and musculoskeletal conditions: A critical review of the literature and proposed methodological standards. Ann Intern Med 1997;127:52–60.
3. Manheim L. Managed care and arthritis care: Patients and providers under the new medical care organizations. Arth Care Res 1995;8:298–303.
4. Yelin E, Trupin L, Katz P. The prevalence and impact of managed care for persons with RA in 1994 and 1999. Arthritis Care Res 2002;47:172–180.
5. Yelin E, Trupin L, Katz P. Impact of managed care on the use of biologic agents for rheumatoid arthritis. Arth Rheum 2005;53:423–430.
6. Yelin E, Trupin L, Katz P, et al. Impact of health maintenance organizations and fee-for-service on health care utilization among people with systemic lupus erythematosus. Arth Care Res 2007;57:508–515.
7. Katz J, Barrett J, Mahomed N, et al. Association between hospital and surgeon procedure volume and outcomes of total knee replacement. J Bone Joint Surg Am 2004;86-A:1909–1916.
8. Katz J, Mahomed N, Baron J, et al. Association of hospital and surgeon procedure volume with patient-centered outcomes of total knee replacement in a population-based cohort of patients age 65 years and older. Arthritis Rheum 2007;56:568–574.
9. Katz J, Bierbaum B, Losina E. Case mix and outcomes of total knee replacement in orthopaedic specialty hospitals. Med Care 2008;46:476–480.
10. Ward M. Association between physician volume and in-hospital mortality in patients with systemic lupus erythematosus. Arth Rheum 2005;52:1646–1654.
11. Hawker G, Wright J, Coyte P, et al. Differences between men and women in the rate of use of hip and knee arthroplasty. N Engl J Med 2000;342:1016–1022.
12. Escalante A, Barrett J, del Rincon I, et al. Disparities between Hispanic and non-Hispanic Medicare beneficiaries in the utilization of total hip replacement. Med Care 2002;40:451–460.

13. Dunlop D, Song J, Manheim L, Chang R. Racial disparities in joint replacement use among older adults. Med Care 2003;41:288–298.

14. Groeneveld P, Kwoh C, Mor M, et al. Racial differences in expectations of joint replacement surgery outcomes. Arthritis Rheum 2008;59:730–737.

15. Dunlop D, Manheim L, Song J, et al. Age and racial/ethnic disparities in arthritis-related hip and knee surgeries. Med Care 2008;46:200–208.

16. Byrne M, O'Malley K, Suarez-Almazor M. Ethnic differences in health preferences: analysis using willingness-to-pay. J Rheumatol 2004;31:1811–1818.

17. Hawker G, Wright J, Badley E, et al. Perceptions of, and willingness to consider, total joint arthroplasty in a population-based cohort of individuals with disabling hip and knee arthritis. Arth Rheum 2004;51:635–641.

18. Hawker G. The quest for explanations for race/ethnic disparity in rates of use of total joint arthroplasty. J Rheumatol 2004;31:1683–1685.

19. Losina E, Barrett J, Baron J, et al. Utilization of low-volume hospitals for total hip replacement. Arthritis Rheum 2004;51:836–842.

20. Fries J, Spitz P, Kraines R, et al. Measurement of patient outcome in arthritis. Arthritis Rheum 1980;23:137–145.

21. Meenan R, Gertman P, Mason J. Measuring health status in arthritis. The arthritis impact measurement scales. Arthritis Rheum 1980;23:146–152.

22. Wolfe F, Michaud K, Pincus T. Development and validation of the health assessment questionaire II: A revised version of the health assessment questionaire. Arthritis Rheum 2004;50:3296–3305.

23. Katz PP, Yelin EH. Life activities of persons with rheumatoid arthritis with and without depressive symptoms. Arthritis Care Res 1994;7:69–77.

24. Meenan R, Yelin E, Henke C, et al. The costs of rheumatoid arthritis. A patient-oriented study of chronic disease costs. Arthritis Rheum 1978;21:827–833.

25. Gibofsky A, Palmer W, Goldman J, et al. Real-world utilization of DMARDs and biologics in rheumatoid arthritis: The RADIUS (Rheumatoid Arthritis Disease-Modifying Anti-Rheumatic Drug Intervention and Utilization Study) study. Curr Med Res Opin 2006;22:169–183.

26. Verstappen S, Jacobs J, Kruize A, et al. Trends in economic consequences of rheumatoid arthritis over two subsequent years. Rheumatology (Oxford) 2007;46:968–974.

27. Rice D. Estimating the cost of illness. Hyattsville, MD: National Center for Health Statistics, Health Economic Series; 1966: No. 6.

28. Rice D, Hodgson T, Kopstein A. The economic costs of illness: A replication and update. Health Care Fin Rev 1985;7:61–80.

29. Rice D. The Economic Burden of Musculoskeletal Conditions, 1995. In: Musculoskeletal Conditions in the United States (Praemer A, Furner S, Rice D, eds.). Rosemont, IL: American Academy of Orthopaedic Surgeons; 1999.

30. Yelin E, Murphy L, Cisternas MG, et al. Medical care expenditures and earnings losses among persons with arthritis and other rheumatic conditions in 2003, and comparisons with 1997. Arthritis Rheum 2007;56:1397–1407.

31. Verbrugge L. Longer life but worsening health? Trends in health and mortality of middle ages and older persons. The Milbank Memorial Fund Quarterly. Health and Society 1984;62:475–519.

32. Verbrugge L, Patrick D. Seven chronic conditions: Their impact on US adults' activity levels and use of medical services. Am J Public Health 1995;85:173–182.

33. Yelin E, Henke C, Epstein W. Resources for the care of arthritics in a non-metropolitan community. Arthritis Rheum 1977;20:45–57.

34. Starr P. The Social Transformation of American Medicine. New York: Basic Books, Inc.; 1982.

35. Lurie I, Dunlop D, Manheim L. Trends in out-of-pocket medica care expenditures for Medicare-age adults with arthritis between 1998 and 2004. Arth Rheum 2008;58:2236–2240.

*Chapter* 17

# The Impact of Technologies on Organization and Progress of Rheumatology Research

**Lars Klareskog**

*Karolinska University Hospital, Rheumatology Unit, Stockholm, Sweden*

**Gerd-Rüdiger Burmester**

*Department of Rheumatology and Clinical Immunology, Charité–University Medicine Berlin, Berlin, Germany*

**Tom W.J. Huizinga**

*Department of Rheumatology, Leiden University Medical Center, Leiden, The Netherlands*

## 17.1 INTRODUCTION

Scientific progress is the most important driver for changes in health care, and in rheumatology, this power has been particularly prominent during the last decade. Technologies are the most decisive power that determines what is possible in science. The challenge is to understand the potentials of these technologies and to create a scientific enterprise that encourages the uptake of new technologies by creative

*The ACR at 75: A Diamond Jubilee*
Copyright © 2009 by John Wiley & Sons, Inc.

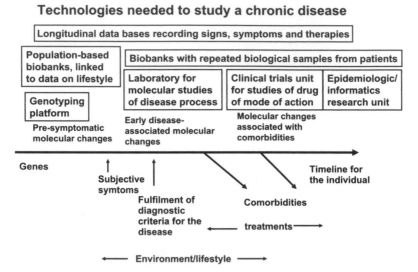

**FIGURE 17.1.** *Illustration of a typical longitudinal course of a chronic rheumatic disease. Below the time line is shown the various clinical events that need to be captured and quantified. Within the squares in the upper part of the figure, we describe technologies that are essential for our understanding of the origins of the disease and for our abilities to influence its outcomes by means of prevention or therapy.*

individuals, to organize science so that technologies and creativity can meet, and to integrate science and health care so that the results of the research enterprise are transformed into clinical practice and public health actions. This chapter aims to describe the progress, potentials, and challenges in technology development in the field of rheumatology (Figure 17.1).

## 17.2  FROM DESCRIPTION OF ILLNESS VIA DEFINITION OF SYNDROMES TOWARDS UNDERSTANDING THE MOLECULAR BASIS OF DISEASE

An important fundamental of clinical medicine is the systematic description of illness and determining critically which recognizable disease features, such as signs (observed by a physician), symptoms (reported by the patient), laboratory phenomena or X-ray characteristics, occur together. Such work provided the foundation for the definition of many of the diseases we know today, and the classical American College of Rheumatology (ACR) criteria for rheumatoid arthritis (RA), Systemic Lupus Erythematosus (SLE) and other diseases are hallmarks of past work and success of rheumatology in this field [1]. Although these classification criteria were constructed from an analysis of relatively few patients and without a goal to reflect a uniform etiology or molecular pathogenesis, they have served us well in identifying conditions (syndromes) sufficiently homogeneous for prediction of disease course and conduct of therapeutic trials.

The challenge of today, however, is different. New technologies now enable us to identify different molecular processes that can be claimed to represent new disease entities, which can cause the signs, symptoms, and other features that qualify for inclusion in a criterion-based syndrome. The challenge in rheumatology and many other disciplines is thus similar to the classic problem in infectious diseases, in which the combined identification of an infectious agent and certain clinical features constitutes the definition of a disease. By analogy, to develop new and useful definitions of disease entities, we need to identify etiologic risk factors (genes and environment), their interactions with disease-associated molecular events, and the way in which symptoms occur. If successful, this work will enable preventive efforts as well as development and testing of both new and old targeted therapies for early use in well-defined groups of patients.

## 17.3 ORIGINS AND OUTCOMES OF ILLNESSS—THE TECHNOLOGIES OF CLINICAL DATA BASES

The classic basis for understanding the origins and outcomes of illness is the longitudinal and quantified documentation of patient signs and symptoms combined with the capture of patient-derived data on lifestyle and environmental exposures that precede and accompany occurrence of the illness. Making this description in an almost infinite number of patients using electronic patient records and data bases is currently revolutionizing our ability to identify the causes of disease (genes and environment) in subsets of the criterion-based syndromes/diseases, and to link both symptoms and effects of treatments to molecular events.

The potentials of these tools to allow primary prevention are demonstrated from identification of lifestyle and environmental causes of disease. Important examples are the roles of smoking, which causes approximately 25% of RA cases in many countries in the world [2], obesity in osteoarthritis [3], and sun exposure in dermatomyositis [4]. The potentials for secondary prevention are particularly obvious in inflammatory rheumatic diseases in which cardiovascular disease [5] as well as lymphomas [6] may result from uninterrupted inflammatory activity and may be preventable by efficient anti-inflammatory treatment.

The potentials for surveillance of effects, adverse effects, and cost-effectiveness of medications and other interventions are also significant. Here, past progress in defining techniques (individual response criteria [7,8]) to determine the response to therapy in individuals rather than in groups has been instrumental for the design of efficient trials of new medications [9]. The challenge is now to use these tools to study the effects of one medication in a disease defined by clinical criteria as well as to investigate and compare complex therapeutic strategies in longitudinal cohorts of patients, who have been categorized with the new tools for analyzing etiology and molecular pathogenesis.

An additional example of the power of longitudinal data bases is illustrated by their successful use in surveillance of adverse drug effects during tumor necrosis factor (TNF)-blockade. Here, the demonstration of a strong increase in the risk for tuberculosis and a moderate increase in risk for other infections has has allowed the more safe use of these drugs [10]. The belated demonstration of cardiovascular adverse events after theuse of rofecoxib and other nonsteroidal anti-inflammatory drugs NSAIDs, however, demonstrates, the consequences of a lack of use of such data bases [11].

The overall challenge now is to organize the capture of relevant and quantifiable information of symptoms and signs from large numbers of patients in clinical practice and make such information available in both the daily encounter between patient and physician and in research. So far, the medical community, including rheumatology, has been slow in embracing the shift from collection of information necessary only for the daily care of small groups of individuals into the modern informatics world. In the modern world, patient-derived information from large groups of patients can be integrated into reclassification of diseases, into studies of etiology, molecular pathogenesis, as well as development and use of new targeted therapies. A change of paradigm has so far occurred mainly regionally and in a few cases, nationally, but it has not reached the general use in medical practice.

## 17.4   UNDERSTANDING DISEASES AND THEIR MOLECULAR MECHANISMS

Today we are witnessing a revolution in the potentials to understand and modulate molecular events in cells as well as in entire organisms. The descriptions of effects of variations in the entire genome [12] is one prime example; the ability to describe the activation of defined pathogenic pathways, such as the α-interferon-dependent signature by global analysis of messenger RNA (mRNA), is another [13,14]. Notably, the identification of molecular pathways responsible for disease development can be immediately followed by efforts aimed at modulating these pathways. Thus, biotechnology now enables the production of almost all molecules that can be produced by mammals, bacteria, and so on, which, in turn, permits interference with almost all processes of life (using monoclonal antibodies, receptor constructs, inhibitory DNA, etc.).

Now, we must combine the potential for molecular understanding and interference with the complex nature of human illness. This effort will require the combination of the clinical and epidemiological science that relies on medical informatics and large data bases with the world of molecular science. Thus, information on environmental and lifestyle factors needs to be combined with genetics and molecular and cell biology to understand the etiology and molecular pathways of new subsets of disease. Information on outcomes in large groups of patients, where information on genotypes and biomarkers are known, will allow the definition of relevant subsets of patients where new targeted therapies can be tested and used.

One example of this development is the now widely accepted subdivision of the syndrome RA into two major subsets [defined by presence or absence of anticitrulline antibodies (ACPAs)], in which different environmental agents working in different genetic contexts may trigger the two variants of disease, and in which early treatment may lead to different results in the two disease subsets [15,16]. Another example is the subdivision of SLE depending on the presence or absence of $\alpha$-interferon activity; in this situation, disease subsets may have different pathogenetic mechanisms and thus be subject to different strategies for development of new therapies [13,14]. Several other examples of this combined use of genetic epidemiology and molecular medicine exist and more will follow.

## 17.5 CONCLUDING REMARKS

Technologies for science are growing with an unprecedented speed, whereas the organization and preparedness for a coordinated use of these technologies for medical research and implementation in clinical care are often lagging. Rheumatology deals with some of medicine's more complex chronic diseases, and rheumatologists and their organizations have been in the forefront in using new technologies in clinical as well as in molecular research. This chapter argues that new initiatives are now needed to continue a bright tradition and that more coordinated efforts are needed to integrate patient and physician derived data captured in data bases with molecular medicine, including genetics. The figure provides an illustration of this concept. It is also essential that work be accomplished within independent academic and clinical medicine to create a global network of collaboration, which can subsequently work with industry and agencies.

## ACKNOWLEDGMENTS

The authors are active in several European and international networks, where combined use of technologies for clinical surveillance as well as molecular studies are crucial. We are convinced that progress will come most efficiently from collaborative work in such large consortia, with opportunities for creative and small-scale work in groups that have access to information and collaboration from these international networks. The authors in particular want to acknowledge the European union-funded program Autocure, as well as several combined ACR-European League against Rheumatism (EULAR) programs as bases for this work

## REFERENCES

1. Arnett FC, Edworthy SM, Bloch DA, et al. The American Rheumatism Association 1987 revised criteria for the classification of rheumatoid arthritis. Arthritis Rheum 1988;31:315–324.
2. Klareskog L, Padyukov L, Alfredsson L. Smoking as a trigger for inflammatory rheumatic diseases. Curr Opin Rheumatol 2007;19:49–54.
3. Berenbaum F, Sellam J. Obesity and osteoarthritis: What are the links? Joint Bone Spine 2008;75:667–668.

4. Okada S, Weatherhead E, Targoff IN, et al. International Myositis Collaborative Study Group. Global surface ultraviolet radiation intensity may modulate the clinical and immunologic expression of autoimmune muscle disease. Arthritis Rheum 2003;48: 2285–2289.

5. Naranjo A, Sokka T, Descalzo MA, et al. QUEST-RA GroupCardiovascular disease in patients with rheumatoid arthritis: Results from the QUEST-RA study. Arthritis Res Ther 2008;10:R30.

6. Baecklund E, Iliadou A, Askling J, et al. Association of chronic inflammation, not its treatment, with increased lymphoma risk in rheumatoid arthritis. Arthritis Rheum 2006;54:692–701.

7. Paulus HE, Egger MJ, Ward JR, et al. Analysis of improvement in individual rheumatoid arthritis patients treated with disease-modifying antirheumatic drugs, based on the findings in patients treated with placebo. The Cooperative Systematic Studies of Rheumatic Diseases Group. Arthritis Rheum 1990;33:477–484.

8. Aletaha D, Landewe R, Karonitsch T, et al. EULAR; ACR. Reporting disease activity in clinical trials of patients with rheumatoid arthritis: EULAR/ACR collaborative recommendations. Arthritis Rheum 2008;59:1371–1377.

9. Elliott MJ, Maini RN, Feldmann M, et al. Randomised double-blind comparison of chimeric monoclonal antibody to tumour necrosis factor alpha (cA2) versus placebo in rheumatoid arthritis. Lancet 1994;344:1105–1110.

10. Zink A, Askling J, Dixon WG, et al. European biologics registers—methodology, selected results, and perspectives. Ann Rheum Dis 2008.

11. Psaty BM, Furberg CD. COX-2 inhibitors—lessons in drug safety. N Engl J Med 2005;352:1133–1135.

12. The Wellcome Trust Case Control Consortium. Genome-wide association study of 14,000 cases of seven common diseases and 3,000 shared controls Nature 2007;447:661–678.

13. Rönnblom L, Eloranta ML, Alm GV. The type I interferon system in systemic lupus erythematosus. Arthritis Rheum 2006;54:408–420.

14. Baechler EC, Batliwalla FM, Karypis G, et al. Interferon-inducible gene expression signature in peripheral blood cells of patients with severe lupus. Proc Natl Acad Sci U S A. 2003;100:2610–2615.

15. Klareskog L, Stolt P, Lundberg K, et al. A new model for an etiology of rheumatoid arthritis: smoking may trigger HLA-DR (shared epitope)-restricted immune reactions to autoantigens modified by citrullination. Arthritis Rheum 2006;54:38–46.

16. van Dongen H, van Aken J, Lard LR, et al. Efficacy of methotrexate treatment in patients with probable rheumatoid arthritis: A double-blind, randomized, placebo-controlled trial. Arthritis Rheum 2007;56:1424–1432.

# Chapter 18

# Genetics of the Rheumatic Diseases in the New Millennium: A New World Emerges

**Peter K. Gregersen**

*Feinstein Institute Medical Research, Genomics and Human Genetics, Manhasset, NY*

## 18.1  IMMUNOGENETICS AND HLA

I began my fellowship training in rheumatology in 1981 at a newly established training program at the Hospital for Joint Diseases in New York City, directed by Dr. Robert Winchester. At that time, the major histocompatibility complex (MHC) was accepted as the most important genetic region involved in controlling the immune response. This was first shown in rodents in work that led to the Nobel Prize in 1980 [1]. However, the state of knowledge about the exact structure and function of the relevant loci in the MHC was limited, and particularly in the human, even the number of genes was not well established. Through the use of serological and cellular typing methods, it was obvious that human leukocyte antigen (HLA) molecules were highly variable in structure (polymorphic), and the molecular basis of this variability was clearly an important problem to tackle. Furthermore, the molecular techniques

*The ACR at 75: A Diamond Jubilee*
Copyright © 2009 by John Wiley & Sons, Inc.

for cloning and sequencing genes were just becoming accessible even to neophytes like me. I was given the opportunity to learn these methods with Dr. Jack Silver (then at Michigan State), who subsequently moved his laboratory to the Hospital for Joint Diseases.

The combination of Bob Winchester's support and longstanding interest in the human HLA system and its relation to human disease, along with Jack Silver's insight and guidance, proved to be an extraordinarily fortunate and productive combination.

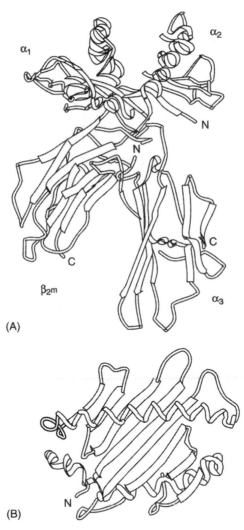

**FIGURE 18.1.** *The X-ray crystallographic structure of an HLA class 1 molecule, which was first reported in 1987 by Bjorkman et al. [3]. Panel A shows the molecule viewed from the side, with the peptide binding cleft at the top of the molecule. The view of this cleft from above is shown in panel B. This structure galvanized the immunological community and permitted a more rational approach to interpreting the flood of genetic information on HLA diversity that emerged in the 1980s and 1990s.*

Among the many ingredients of scientific success, luck and being in the right place at the right time were clearly important. The other essential ingredient was persistence. The techniques of complementary DNA (cDNA) cloning and sequencing were slow and painstaking at the time, very crude in comparison with today's off-the-shelf approach. It took me 4 years to publish my first major paper reporting on the molecular diversity of DR4 alleles [2], but that experience made it obvious to me that I wanted to be a full-time scientist.

During the 1980's, dramatic advances were achieved in the field of immunogenetics. Many major HLA alleles were sequenced, and the structure of an HLA molecule worked out by Pamela Bjorkman and Don Wiley [3] became iconic (Figure 18.1). Suddenly, a three-dimensional structure was available which we could map all these new polymorphisms. The sense of optimism at that time was palpable. Toward the end of the 1980s, a seminal figure in the field was quoted in the *New York Times* [4]: "We're within a gnat's hair of understanding everything we need to know about how the immune system reacts." Of course, in retrospect, this seems naïve, but it catches the thrill of new discovery that many of us experienced at the time.

## 18.2  THE 1990'S — FILLING IN THE DETAILS AND LAYING FOUNDATIONS

Using the new sequenced-based HLA typing, a much more precise approach to disease association in the rheumatic diseases became possible. For example, the association of the shared epitope sequence with rheumatoid arthritis (RA) was confirmed and refined [5,6], and the HLA associations in lupus, Sjogren's Syndrome, and other autoimmune diseases were clearly shown to relate primarily to the production of particular autoantibody specificities [7,8]; this theme has now reemerged in the study of anticitrulline antibodies in RA [9]. Work in basic immunology continued to reveal the molecular details of peptide binding and T-cell interactions with the HLA molecules, providing the basis for hypotheses about the underlying cause of these associations (a problem that has yet to be fully solved, gnat hairs notwithstanding!).

However, as the decade progressed, many investigators began to think ahead about how to identify genes outside of the MHC that might be involved in autoimmunity. John Harley, Tim Behrens, Mike Seldin, and Dan Kastner were among the small group of rheumatologists who regularly put in an appearance at the annual meeting of the American Society of Human Genetics. The development of panels of "microsatellite" markers [10], which are based on the presence of large numbers of loci in the genome with variable numbers of tandem repeats (VNTRs), generated excitement in the field for applying linkage analysis to rheumatic disorders. Linkage analysis depends on collecting large numbers of multiplex families or affected siblings with a disease or trait, and it is most valuable for studying traits with a clear Mendelian pattern (dominant or recessive) of inheritance. Linkage analysis was remarkably successful in leading to the identification of the gene for Familial Mediterranean Fever by Dan Kastner and colleagues in 1997 [11]. The identification of genes for several other autoinflammatory disorders followed [12], and by 2000, the genetic discovery for this group of disorders became a major success story.

Considerable skepticism (with some justification) existed about the utility of applying linkage approaches to more complex disorder, such as lupus or rheumatoid arthritis. Nonetheless, optimism prevailed, and collections of multiplex families and/ or affected sibling pairs were assembled to carry out linkage studies of both RA and lupus. As it turns out, the genetic basis of many rheumatic diseases has proved to be far more complex than originally anticipated, and in general, linkage has been a disappointing method for gene identification in the more common, non-Mendelian rheumatic diseases. Nevertheless, linkage analysis has led to the identification of a few genes for some complex autoimmune diseases, such as the NOD2 locus in Crohn's disease [13,14], and more recently STAT4 in rheumatoid arthritis and lupus [15]. More importantly, the availability of these large DNA collections of patients and families became invaluable for subsequent association studies and particularly for the large scale genome wide association studies that have been so productive in recent years.

## 18.3  THE NEW MILLENNIUM: GENOME WIDE ASSOCIATION STUDIES (GWAS) AND BEYOND

The completion of the Human Genome Project in 2001 has ushered in a new era in human genetics [16]; however, the International HapMap project has been an equally important catalyst for mapping human disease [17]. The HapMap is a large collaborative international effort to define the sequence diversity in human populations, with an emphasis on relatively common genetic variation in the form of single nucleotide polymorphsism (SNPs). Any two unrelated individuals in the population are likely to differ by about 0.1% across the genome of $\sim$3.2 billion base pairs, or approximately 3 million SNP differences. The HapMap also established the patterns of linkage disequilibrium among these SNPs, forming common haplotypes (groups of adjacent SNP alleles running together in the population) that exist within the three major racial groups — Caucasian, Asian, and African. This led to the realization that a large proportion of the common differences between any two individuals can be captured by looking at 300—500,000 SNPs across the genome, rather than having to genotype all 3 million SNP differences. The HapMap is an extraordinarily interesting, powerful, and useful scientific resource. It is easily accessible on the web (http://www. hapmap.org/) and is well worth a visit even for nongeneticists to learn about its history and experience the various visualization tools that capture patterns of common variation across the human genome.

The HapMap is important because it has allowed for the intelligent design and interpretation of a "genome-wide" approach to disease association. During the 1990s and the early part of the new millennium, virtually all genetic association studies were carried out to examine "candidate" genes (e.g., genes for which a plausible hypothesis was developed based on limited biological knowledge). This new genome-wide approach is an example of "discovery-driven" science, in which tens or hundreds of thousands of hypotheses are tested simultaneously. Initially, this approach to investigation was met with a good deal of skepticism [18]. A common concern, even among geneticists, was that if you perform enough tests you are going to find something, but does it mean anything? Nevertheless, beginning with a dramatic success in mapping genes for macular degeneration [19], genome-wide association studies have been remarkably successful in finding new genes underlying complex human diseases and perhaps nowhere more so than in the field of rheumatic and autoimmune disorders [20,21].

Writing now in late 2008, it is clear that we are still in the middle of a revolution in our understanding of the genetics of rheumatic diseases. However, several themes are emerging. First, most common rheumatic and autoimmune disorders have a genetic component that involves many genes — certainly on the order of 20–50 genes and perhaps more [22]. Each of these new risk variants contributes a relatively modest degree of risk, generally twofold or less. Second, it is now abundantly clear that many of these newly discovered genetic variants contribute to risk for several different autoimmune disorders, sometimes in contrasting ways. A good example is the intracellular phosphatase PTPN22 [23] in which an amino acid substitution of tryptophan for arginine at codon 620 confers risk for rheumatoid arthritis, type 1 diabetes, autoimmune thyroid disease, lupus, and myasthenia gravis, to name a few. However this polymorphism provides no risk for multiple sclerosis, and in fact it is protective for Crohn's Disease [22]. Thus, the data are showing that autoimmune diseases fall into groups of disorders that share, or are distinguished by, specific pathways of pathogenesis [20,21]. This major advance is likely to be translated into new diagnostics and therapeutics in the coming decade.

Finally, new concepts and insights continue to emerge about the genetic architecture of human disease generally, including rheumatic disorders. The current wave of discovery has been almost entirely focused on the common genetic variants (e.g., genetic variation which has generally been selected in the course of human evolution to favor survival). Thus, a proportion of disease burden in the current population reflects the price we pay for the survival our ancestors. However, we are still left with a considerable amount of "missing heritability", and it seems likely that another component of the genetic burden for disease involves relatively rare and perhaps more recent genetic variation — the TREX1 associations with lupus may be an example of this [24]. Furthermore, it is now apparent that large-scale structural variation in the genome is occurring frequently; a significant fraction of normal offspring seem to have large changes in their genomes — deletions or duplications — that are not present in either parent [25]. Monozygotic twins, which were previously thought to always be absolutely genetically identical, have now occasionally been shown to have significant genetic differences between them [26]. Beyond these unexpected findings, epigenetic variation (DNA methylation and histone modification) has just begun to be investigated as a potential source of phenotypic variability. These observations suggest to me that the next 25 years of research on the genetics of rheumatic disease are likely to be surprising and transforming, far more so than the last 25 years. I hope to continue to participate actively and contribute to this evolving story.

## REFERENCES

1. Benacerraf B. Role of MHC gene products in immune regulation. Science 1981; 212:1229–1238.
2. Gregersen PK, Shen M, Song QL, et al. Molecular diversity of HLA-DR4 haplotypes. Proc Natl Acad Sci U S A 1986;83:2642–2646.
3. Bjorkman PJ, Saper MA, Samraoui B, et al. Structure of the human class I histocompatibility antigen, HLA-A2. Nature 1987;329:506–512.
4. Kolata G. New research yields clues in fight against autoimmune diseases. The New York Times 1988 (January 19).
5. Weyand CM, Hicok KC, Conn DL, Goronzy JJ. The influence of HLA-DRB1 genes on disease severity in rheumatoid arthritis. Ann Intern Med 1992;117:801–806.
6. Hall FC, Weeks DE, Camilleri JP, et al. Influence of the HLA-DRB1 locus on susceptibility and severity in rheumatoid arthritis. Qjm 1996;89:821–829.
7. Harley JB, Reichlin M, Arnett FC, et al. Gene interaction at HLA-DQ enhances autoantibody production in primary Sjogren's syndrome. Science 1986;232:1145–1147.
8. Reveille JD, Macleod MJ, Whittington K, Arnett FC. Specific amino acid residues in the second hypervariable region of HLA- DQA1 and DQB1 chain genes promote the Ro (SS-A)/La (SS-B) autoantibody responses. J Immunol 1991;146:3871–3876.
9. Ding B, Padyukov L, Lundstrom E, et al. Different patterns of associations with anti-citrullinated protein antibody-positive and anti-citrullinated protein antibody-negative rheumatoid arthritis in the extended major histocompatibility complex region. Arthritis Rheum 2009;60:30–38.
10. Todd JA. La carte des microsatellites est arrivee! [The map of microsatellites has arrived!]. Hum Mol Genet 1992;1:663–666.
11. Ancient missense mutations in a new member of the RoRet gene family are likely to cause familial Mediterranean fever. The International FMF Consortium. Cell 1997;90:797–807.
12. McDermott MF, Aksentijevich I, Galon J, et al. Germline mutations in the extracellular domains of the 55 kDa TNF receptor, TNFR1, define a family of dominantly inherited autoinflammatory syndromes. Cell 1999;97:133–144.
13. Ogura Y, Bonen DK, Inohara N, et al. A frameshift mutation in NOD2 associated with susceptibility to Crohn's disease. Nature 2001;411:603–606.
14. Hugot JP, Chamaillard M, Zouali H, et al. Association of NOD2 leucine-rich repeat variants with susceptibility to Crohn's disease. Nature 2001;411:599–603.
15. Remmers EF, Plenge RM, Lee AT, et al. STAT4 and the risk of rheumatoid arthritis and systemic lupus erythematosus. N Engl J Med 2007;357:977–986.
16. Lander ES, Linton LM, Birren B, et al. Initial sequencing and analysis of the human genome. Nature 2001;409:860–921.
17. A haplotype map of the human genome. Nature 2005;437:1299–1320.
18. Weiss KM, Terwilliger JD. How many diseases does it take to map a gene with SNPs? Nat Genet 2000;26:151–157.
19. Klein RJ, Zeiss C, Chew EY, et al. Complement factor H polymorphism in age-related macular degeneration. Science 2005;308:385–389.
20. Zhernakova A, van Diemen CC, Wijmenga C. Detecting shared pathogenesis from the shared genetics of immune-related diseases. Nat Rev Genet 2009;10:43–55.

21. Gregersen PK, Olsson LM. Recent advances in the genetics of autoimmune disease. Ann Rev Immun 2009;27:363–391.

22. Barrett JC, Hansoul S, Nicolae DL, et al. Genome-wide association defines more than 30 distinct susceptibility loci for Crohn's disease. Nat Genet 2008;40:955–962.

23. Gregersen PK, Lee HS, Batliwalla F, Begovich AB. PTPN22: Setting thresholds for autoimmunity. Semin Immunol 2006;18:214–223.

24. Lee- Kirsch MA, Gong M, Chowdhury D, et al. Mutations in the gene encoding the 3′-5′ DNA exonuclease TREX1 are associated with systemic lupus erythematosus. Nat Genet 2007;39:1065–1067.

25. Sebat J, Lakshmi B, Malhotra D, et al. Strong association of de novo copy number mutations with autism. Science 2007;316:445–449.

26. Bruder CE, Piotrowski A, Gijsbers AA, et al. Phenotypically concordant and discordant monozygotic twins display different DNA copy-number-variation profiles. Am J Hum Genet 2008;82:763–771.

**PROGRAM**

# Conference on Rheumatic Diseases

AN OPEN MEETING SPONSORED BY

## The American Committee for the Control of Rheumatism

**MONDAY, MAY 9, 1932, NINE O'CLOCK A.M. TO TWELVE NOON**

**Hotel Roosevelt, Room A, New Orleans**

---

It is requested that papers be presented in abstract, not read. Time limit for papers will be 12 minutes. (For total discussion of any one paper time limit 8 minutes). Discussions of any paper by members of the audience are cordially invited.

---

1. Chairman's Introduction—Dr. Ralph Pemberton, Philadelphia

2. "Clinical and Economic Factors of Arthritis in 450 Ex-members of the Military Service.".........
.........................Dr. Philip B. Matz, Washington, D. C.

   Discussion: Dr. Wallace S. Duncan, Cleveland, Ohio, and Dr. Francis C. Hall, Boston.

3. "Relation of the Digestive Tract to Chronic Arthritis"
   ...........Dr. T. Preston White, Charlotte, North Carolina

4. "Gallbladder Disease in Chronic Infectious Arthritis: Results of Cholecystectomy"..............Dr. E. Starr Judd (and Dr. Philip S. Hench), Rochester, Minnesota

   Discussion (papers No. 3 and No. 4): Dr. R. Garfield Snyder, New York City, and Dr. A. R. Shands, Jr., Durham, North Carolina.

(a)

*Program of the first meeting.*

5. "Climate Therapy for Chronic Arthritis: Results in 500 Cases"..............Dr. W. Paul Holbrook, Tucson, Arizona

6. "The Desensitization Treatment of Chronic Arthritis"............Dr. James Craig Small, Philadelphia

7. "Intravenous Streptococcic Vaccine Therapy in Chronic Arthritis"............Dr. Macnider Wetherby, Minneapolis

   Discussion (papers No. 5, No. 6 and No. 7) : Dr. John W. Gray, Newark, New Jersey; Dr. Wm. J. Kerr, San Francisco, California, and Dr. O. O. Ashworth, Richmond, Virginia

*Papers to be read if time permits*

8. "Sinus Infections as Silent Foci in Arthritis"........ ..................................Dr. R. Garfield Snyder, New York

9. "Degenerative Arthritis in Ilio-femoral Ligaments"....................Dr. Edward K. Cravener, Boston

10. "The Joints in Infection"........Dr. Chester S. Keefer, and Dr. Walter K. Meyers, Boston ........................ .... .. .. ......

11. "The Arthritis Problem"........Dr. Millard Smith, Boston

12. "Classification of Osteo-arthritis"............................. ............................Dr. Walter Gay Lough, New York City

---

You are cordially invited to visit the exhibit of the **American Committee for The Control of Rheumatism** to be held in Booths **1004, 1006, 1008** and **1010** in the **Exhibit Hall.**

Ralph Pemberton, M. D., Philadelphia, *Chairman*
Charles C. Bass, M. D., New Orleans
Russell L. Cecil, M. D., New York
A. Almon Fletcher, M. D., Toronto
Russell L. Haden, M. D., Cleveland
Melvin S. Henderson, M. D., Rochester, Minnesota

Joseph L. Miller, M. D., Chicago
George R. Minot, M. D., Boston
J. Archer O'Reilly, M. D., St. Louis
Robert B. Osgood, M. D., Boston
Cyrus C. Sturgis, M. D., Ann Arbor
Hans Zinsser, M. D., Boston
Philip S. Hench, M. D., Rochester, Minnesota, *Secretary*

(b)

*Program of the first meeting.*

American Committee for Control of Rheumatism 1928-1934
Scientific Meetings 1932-1934
Ralph Pemberton, Chairman

American Association for the Study and Control of Rheumatic Diseases 1934-1937

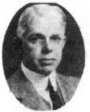
Emest F. Irons
1934–35

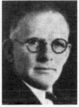
Russell L. Haden
1935–36

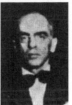
Russell L. Cecil
1936–37

American Rheumatism Association 1937-1960

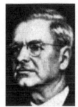
William J. Kerr
1937–38

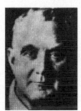
Ralph Pemberton
1938–39

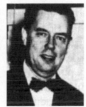
Philip C. Hench
1939–40

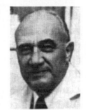
Ralph H. Boots
1940–41

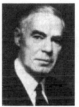
Loring T. Swain
1941–42

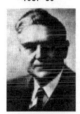
W. Paul Holbrook
1942–45

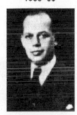
Walter Bauer
1946–47

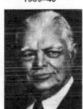
Robert M. Stecher
1947–48

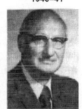
Richard H. Freyberg
1948–49

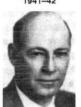
T. Duckett Jones
1949–50

Otto Steinbroker
1950–51

Charles H. Slocumb
1951–52

Currier McEwen
1952–53

Charles Ragan
1953–54

Edward W. Boland
1954–55

Charles L. Short
1955–56

William D. Robinson
1956–57

L. Maxwell Lockie
1957–58

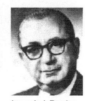
Joseph J. Bunim
1958–59

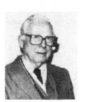
Charley J. Smyth
1959–60

*Leadership (1928–1960).*

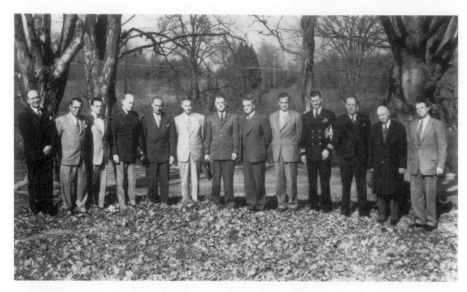

First Meeting of the National Advisory Arthritis and Metabolic Diseases Council, November 15, 1950, Dr. William H. Sebrell, Jr., Dr. John A. Reed, Dr. Maxwell Wintrobe, Col. Paul S. Fancher, Dr. Richard H. Freyberg, Dr. Cecil J. Watson, Lt. Co. William D. Preston, Dr. W. Paul Holbrook, Dr. Alfred H. Lawton, Cmdr. J.S. Cowan, Mr. Wrston Howland, Mr. Clyde E. Wildman, and Dr. Floyd S. Draft.

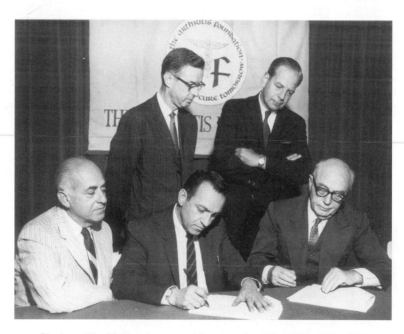

Signing of the Merger Agreement between the AF and the ARA, 1965.

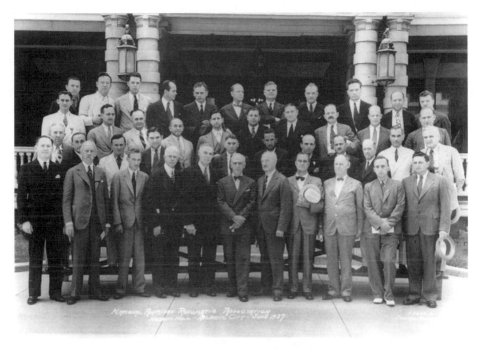

*National American Rheumatic Association, Atlantic City, June 1937.*

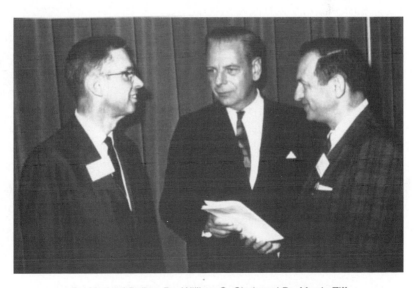

*Dr. Howard Polley, Dr. William S, Clark and Dr. Morris Ziff.*

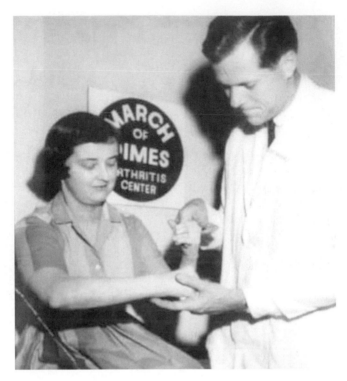

*Dr. Charles Christian with a patient.*

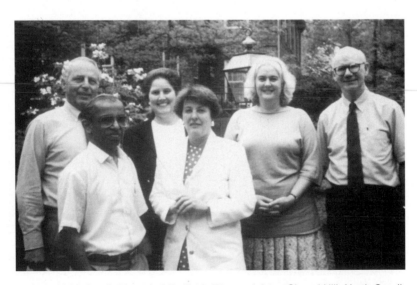

*Members of the first Subboard of Pediatric Rheumatology, Chapel Hill, North Carolina.*

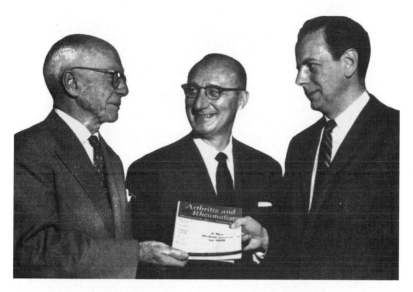

*Publication of the First Issue of A&R, Dr. Russell Cecil, Dr. Richard Freyburg, and Dr. William Clark, 1958.*

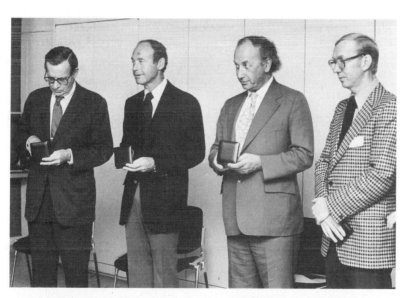

*August 1978. First International Congress on Inflammation held to celebrate the 900$^{th}$ Anniversary of the founding of the University of Bologna. Shown are Drs. Lewis Thomas, Gerald Weissmann, John Vane and Bengt Samuelsson, receiving the Gold Medal of the University of Bologna.*

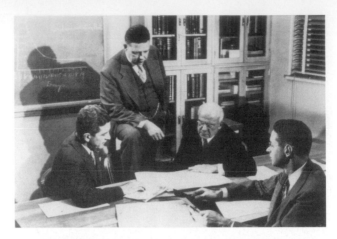

*The Cortisone Story, 1949, Charles H. Slocumb, MD, Philip S. Hench, MD,   E.G. Kendall, MD, and Howard F. Polley, MD.*

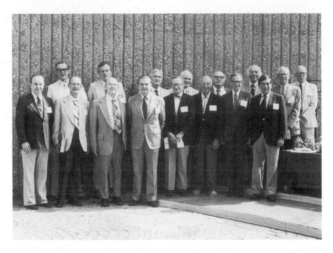

*ACR Past Presidents, 1980, Dr. Carl Pearson, Dr. John Decker, Dr. William Robertson, Dr. Joe Hollander, Dr. Chuck Christian, Dr. Edward Boland, Dr. Emmerson Ward, Dr. Alan Cohen, Dr. Daniel McCarty, Dr. Richard Freyburg, Dr. Gerald Rodnan, Dr. Morris Ziff, Dr. Ephraim Engleman, Dr. Lawrence Shulman, Dr. McEwen, and Dr. Charlie Smuth.*

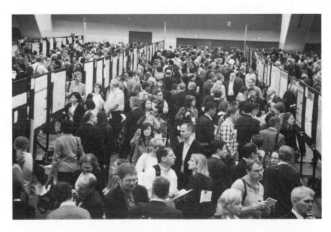

*2008 Annual Scientific Meeting.*

# Chapter 19

# A Revolution
# in Immunology

**Gerald Weissmann**

*New York University Medical Center, Department of Medicine, New York, NY*

## 19.1   A REVOLUTION IN IMMUNOLOGY

Rheumatology came late to the game of medical science and even later to immunology. From 1933 to 1948, our medical specialty was a descriptive art; in any meaningful way, we had no idea of what was going on. Cardiologists had their electrocardiography (EKGs) and digitalis, and the endocrinologists had their thyroid tests and extracts, but rheumatologists seemed condemned to stand idly by to watch their patients turn into cripples or die in lupus crisis after one or another stopgap treatments. Oh yes, we had diathermy, gold salts, paraffin injections and, believe it or not, bee venom. We knew how to treat gout with colchicine, were just learning to give penicillin to prevent rheumatic fever, but by and large, our treatment of joint disease or even Systemic Lupus Erythematosus (SLE) was limited to aspirin, aspirin, and more aspirin. All that changed in the *annus mirabilus* of our field, 1948.

At a staff meeting of the Mayo Clinic in January of 1948, Malcolm M. Hargraves described a strange kind of cell that formed in blood samples of patients with SLE [1]. Before 1950, we could not really tell who had SLE and who did not; we had no clue as why it was so often fatal. Hargraves has discovered what he called the LE cell, which finally not only permitted us to make a diagnosis of the disease but also told us what was going wrong with these poor women. The LE cell, it turned out over the years, is a white blood cell (a neutrophil) that has ingested the dying nucleus of another cell against which lupus patients make antibodies. Complement was involved, which acted as an opsonin. It also turned out that those antibodies against the nucleus and/or its constituents—the anti-DNA antibodies—were just the tip of an iceberg. SLE patients make a dazzling number of antibodies with their Fab regions directed against bits and pieces of their own cells. Their immune system recognizes such bits of "self" as if they were a microbe, which is a tad of "non-self" that wants expunging. Hargrave's discovery of the LE cell sparked the study of autoimmunity and lifted rheumatology over the threshold of science [1].

In the same month, immunologist Harry Rose and rheumatologist Charles Ragan of Columbia described a factor in the serum of most patients with rheumatoid arthritis (RA) that clumped sheep red blood cells coated with human antibodies: the "sensitized sheep cell agglutination test" [2]. Tests for this factor not only permitted accurate diagnosis of rheumatoid arthritis but also taught us how joints are attacked in RA. What came to be called the "rheumatoid factor" turned out to be yet another autoantibody, which was of great size and with a tendency to form sludge in the blood. Normal human antibodies, the "self" in this case, were recognized as "non-self" by rheumatoid factor. The agglutination reaction in a test tube was a pretty good reflection of what happens in life. In patients with RA, complexes of antibodies that contain rheumatoid factor form in the blood like *iles flottant*; they become trapped in joint spaces, joint cells try to get rid of the unwanted debris, cry havoc and let loose the dogs of inflammation: anaphylatoxins C3a, C5a, eicosanoids, and so on. As with Hargraves and the LE cell, the discovery of rheumatoid factor made it possible to make sense of yet one more of our diseases. RA is an immune complex disease, in which complement is activated, as Peter Ward and Nathan Zvaifler were the first to document [3].

On April 20, 1949, William A. Lawrence of *The New York Times* broke news of another discovery announced at a staff meeting at the Mayo Clinic:

> Preliminary tests during the last 7 months at the Mayo Clinic with a hormone from the skin of the adrenal glands has opened up an entirely new approach to the treatment of rheumatoid arthritis, the most painful form of arthritis, that cripples millions, it was revealed here tonight, [3].

That evening, Philip Hench, Charles Slocumb, and Howard Polley reported their experience with 14 cases of rheumatoid arthritis treated with a precious material called "Kendall's compound E" or 17 hydroxy-11 dehydro-corticosterone [4]. Cortisone had entered the clinic.

Within a week, cinemas nationwide showed newsreels of cripples rising miraculously from their wheelchairs. By May 1949, Hench and coworkers reported the "complete remission of acute signs and symptoms of rheumatoid inflammation" at the Association of American Physicians in Atlantic City. In June, they added success with rheumatic fever to the cortisone legend at the Seventh International Congress of Rheumatic Diseases in New York. It was the summer I decided to follow my father into rheumatology and, in retrospect, I guess that it was cortisone that convinced me.

I will never forget the waves of applause after Hench's dramatic film clips were shown to a packed crowd at the Waldorf Astoria. One could actually *do* something about a crippling disease like rheumatoid arthritis.

In October 1950, the Nobel committee announced that Philip Hench and the two biochemists who had painstakingly isolated and described the chemistry of adrenal steroids, Thaddeus Reichstein (University of Basel) and Edward Kendall (Mayo Clinic), would receive the Nobel Prize in Physiology or Medicine for "their discoveries relating to the hormones of the adrenal cortex, their structure and biological effects" [5]. Hench remains the only rheumatologist among Nobel laureates. So universal was the acclaim for cortisone that the Swedish announcement of the 1950 Nobel prize in literature (William Faulkner) was almost a footnote in the world press [6].

Studies of how cortisone works its magic in rheumatoid arthritis and SLE led two generations of rheumatologists into the field. Their studies have contributed both to the basic science of immunology and to the treatment of patients with rheumatic disease. It must be admitted, however, that nothing we have learned since Hench's Nobel Prize has given us any notion of what *causes* either lupus or rheumatoid arthritis. We have, however, learned much about how immune reactions mediate the pathology of RA and SLE.

Immunoglobulin G (IgG)/IgM complexes have been implicated in RA since the early work in Joseph Hollander's laboratory. He explained the crucial experiments of 1965:

> To test further our hypothesis of the immunopathogenesis of rheumatoid arthritis, we isolated gamma-G from rheumatoid serum and injected a few milligrams of this into an uninflamed knee joint of the patient from whom the serum was obtained. In every case an acute joint inflammation developed within hours, but gamma-G from normal donors, prepared identically and in the same dose, caused no reaction in the contralateral knee at the same time. Rheumatoid gamma-G injected into osteoarthritic joints (seronegative for rheumatoid factor) produced no inflammatory response. [7]

When such complexes are taken up by phagocytes in the joint, they form the "RA cell," which is a cell analogous to the LE cell of Hargraves. The circulating complexes are not specific for RA; they are found in other rheumatic and autoimmune diseases as well as having a low prevalence in the normal population. Recently, other antigens that result in autoimmune complex formation with greater specificity for RA have been described. These antibodies, which are known as anticyclic citrullinated peptide (anti-CCP) antibodies recognize citrullinated protein residues that are present as antigenic determinants in patients with RA [8]. Mart Mannik had earlier found that some 7s IgG rheumatoid factors self-aggregate to form larger immune complexes via hydrophobic interactions to become trapped within the synovial tissue [9].

This is in contrast to SLE, which is another autoimmune disease characterized by immune complexes in the systemic circulation. In the case of SLE, 7s IgGs directed against several nuclear antigens localize mainly in the kidneys and blood vessels [10]. They also produce cerebral and pulmonary disease by activating complement

**TABLE 19.1    Comparison of Immune Complex Formation in the Autoimmune Diseases RA and SLE**

| Immune Response | RA | SLE |
| --- | --- | --- |
| Diagnostic "tell-tale" cell | RA cell (phagocytes with ingested rheumatoid factor complexes) | LE cell (phagocytes with ingested cell nuclei) |
| Antigen | Hinge region of IgG | DNA, histones, etc.; phospholipids |
| Antibody | 19s IgM, self-agg7s IgG | 7s IgG |
| Antigen/antibody deposition | Synovium, cartilage | Kidneys, blood vessels |
| Complement activation | Synovial fluid C3a, C5a, C5b-9 | Systemic C1q, C3a, C5a, C5b-9 |

systemically [11]. Genetic defects in the complement cascade associated with SLE result in inadequate clearance of immune complexes as well as apoptotic blebs containing autoantigens [12].

Table 19.1 summarizes the role of immune complexes in the two diseases. In RA, immune complexes cause local joint inflammation by activating complement and stimulating phagocytes directly. Neutrophils, which comprise more than 90% of the total cell population in synovial fluid, take up immune complexes via Fc receptors that trigger the release of hydrolytic enzymes, the generation of reactive oxygen species, and products of arachidonic acid metabolism. These products promote an inflammatory response and/or lead directly to tissue degradation [13].

We could therefore say that tissue injury in RA is caused by a combination of phagocytosis (innate immunity) and anaphylaxis (acquired immunity) gone awry. Immune complexes create their havoc via Fc gamma III receptors that signal via the tyrosine phosphorylation immunoreceptor pathway. Anaphylatoxins, mainly C5a, signal via the mitogen extracellular kinase (MEK)/mitogen-activated protein (MAP) kinase cascade, and both engage in crosstalk via nuclear factor (NF) kappa B. We now appreciate that cytokines such as tumor necrosis factor (TNF) alpha and interleukin-1 (IL-1) are important mediators of inflammation in RA [14], but in the joint they act downstream of the primary insults: immune complexes and anaphylatoxins. Many of the currently used and developing therapeutic strategies against RA are targeted successfully toward these cytokines, which were first appreciated as "lymphokines" [15]. Others are directed toward the cell–cell interactions between subsets of T cells and B cells—and now of other antigen-presenting cells—that produce the autoantibodies in the first place.

Although we have no clue as to the true etiology of either SLE or RA diseases, we have dramatically changed the treatment of both diseases. The new biologic agents and small molecules that curb rheumatic disease have resulted from decades of basic discovery in made in the laboratory. We owe much to the pioneers of experimental rheumatology who have taught us the basic facts I have outlined here: K Frank Austen, Claude Bennett, Charles Christian, Edward C. Franklin, Joseph Hollander, Halsted Holman, Stephen Krane, Henry Kunkel, Mart Mannik, Steve Malawista, Hans Mueller-Eberhart, Lewis Thomas, John Vaughan, Morris Ziff, and Nathan Zvaifler.

# REFERENCES

1. Hargraves MM, Morton R. Presentation of 2 bone marrow elements—the tart cell and the LE cell Proc Staff M Mayo Clin 1948;23:25–28.

2. Rose HM, Ragan C, Pearce E, et al. Differential agglutination of normal and sensitized sheep erythrocytes by sera of patients with Rheumatoid Arthritis Proc Soc Exp Biol Med 1948;68:1–6.

3. Ward PA, Zvaifler NJ. Complement-derived leukotactic factors in inflammatory synovial fluids of humans. J Clin Invest 1971;50:606–616.

4. Laurence WA. Aid in rheumatoid arthritis is promised by new hormone. New York Times 1949(April 21).

5. Hench PS, Kendall EC, Slocumb CH, et al. The effect of a hormone of the adrenal cortex (17 hydroxy-11 dehydrocorticosterone: compound E) and of pituitary adrenocorticotropic hormone on rheumatoid arthritis. (Preliminary report) Proc Staff Meetings Mayo Clinic 1949;24:181–297.

6. The Nobel Prize in physiology or Medicine 1950. Nobel prize.org. Available at http://www.nobel.se/medicine/laureates/1950.

7. Hollander JL, McCarty DJ, Astorga G, et al. Studies on the pathogenesis of rheumatoid joint inflammation. I. The "R.A. cell" and a working hypothesis. Ann Intern Med 1965;62:271–280.

8. Kroot EJ, de Jong BA, van Leeuwen MA, et al. The prognostic value of anti-cyclic citrullinated peptide antibody in patients with recent-onset rheumatoid arthritis. Arthritis Rheum 2000;43:1831–1835.

9. Pope RM, Teller DC, Mannik M. The molecular basis of self-association of antibodies to IgG (rheumatoid factors) in rheumatoid arthritis. Proc Natl Acad Sci U S A 1974;71:517–521.

10. Atkinson JP. Complement activation and complement receptors in systemic lupus erythematosus. Springer Semin Immunopathol 1986;9:179–194.

11. Belmont HM, Hopkins P, Edelson HS, et al. Complement activation during systemic lupus erythematosus. C3a and C5a anaphylatoxins circulate during exacerbations of disease. Arthritis Rheum 1986;29:1085–1089.

12. Davies KA, Schifferli JA, Walport MJ. Complement deficiency and immune complex disease. Springer Semin Immunopathol 1994;115:397–416.

13. Weissmann G, Zurier RB, Spieler PJ, et al. Mechanisms of lysosomal enzyme release from leukocytes exposed to immune complexes and other particles. J Exp Med 1971;134:149s–156s.

14. Krane SM, Dayer JM, Simon LS, et al. Mononuclear cell-conditioned medium containing mononuclear cell factor (MCF), homologous with interleukin 1, stimulates collagen and fibronectin synthesis by adherent rheumatoid synovial cells: effects of prostaglandin E2 and indomethacin. Coll Relat Res. 1985;5:99–117.

15. Dumonde DC, Wolstencroft RA, Panayi GS, et al. "Lymphokines": Non-antibody mediators of cellular immunity generated by lymphocyte activation. Nature 1969;224:38–42.

# Chapter 20

# *Autoantibodies*

**Eng M. Tan**

*Scripps Research Institute, W M Keck Autoimmune Disease Center, La Jolla, CA*

Clinical and basic research in the study of autoantibodies has been pioneered by the subspecialty of rheumatology. This focus is in part related to the fact that illnesses that are classic examples of autoimmunity, such as systemic lupus erythematosus (SLE), rheumatoid arthritis, Sjogren's syndrome, and progressive systemic sclerosis (scler-oderma), are generally treated by rheumatologists. These illnesses are frequently systemic in nature and involve diverse organs. Interestingly, and perhaps not accidentally, autoantibodies in these rheumatic illnesses are reactive with protein and nucleic acid antigens that are widely distributed in most cell types; these antigens are not restricted to cells of specific organs. With most organ-specific autoimmune diseases, such as type 1 diabetes and multiple sclerosis, the targeted antigens are more restricted to specific organs. This chapter will consider the important contributions of rheumatology in elucidating the nature of autoantibodies and their cognate antigens, as well as the role of autoantibodies as biomarkers and as instruments of disease pathogenesis

## 20.1 DEFINING THE NATURE AND PROPERTIES OF ANTIGENS REACTIVE WITH AUTOANTIBODIES

In the late 1950s and early 1960s, important advances were made in identifying the presence of autoantibodies to DNA and histones in sera of patients with SLE [1,2]. A leading immunologist of that era, Henry G. Kunkel of the Rockefeller University, was one of a handful of scientists who made these observations. In personal memoirs, he noted that the identification of autoantibody to DNA was greeted initially with intense skepticism. However, in his laconic way, he said that this observation was ultimately accepted because he had the facts. This ground-breaking finding may have made others in the field too complacent. Indeed, one investigator at that time proclaimed that there was nothing more to do with autoantibodies in SLE after the discovery of antibody to DNA. He was completely mistaken.

At that time, the Rockefeller University in New York ran a small clinic and hospital, which was funded by the National Institutes of Health in the form of a general clinical research center (GCRC). One of the research projects was a study of SLE, and one of the patients observed there was a young girl named Stephanie Smith. Her serum contained an antibody that was to become the prototype of an antibody to nuclear antigens, which were neither DNA nor histones [3]. At the time of this discovery, little was known about nonhistone nuclear proteins. The antigen defined by the patient's serum antibody is now called the Sm antigen, and the publication of this observation has been selected as one of the Pillars of Immunology by the *Journal of Immunology* [4].

The Sm antibody has played a crucial role in elucidating an important gene transcription pathway in cell biology. The antibody was used to immunoprecipitate intracellular particles that contain the Sm antigen and, in one single step, purified the Sm antigen and other proteins and nucleic acids bound to it. This SLE autoantibody helped elucidate an important cellular mechanism called splicing, which processes precursor messenger RNA into mature messenger RNA [5]. Stephanie Smith, who succumbed to her illness, was a talented artist and left behind several of her oil paintings, which were given to physicians at the Rockefeller University involved in her care.

## 20.2  IMMUNE COMPLEXES OF AUTOANTIBODIES AND ANTIGENS ARE INVOLVED IN PATHOGENESIS

Immunological studies in experimental animals had long indicated the pathogenic potential of antigen–antibody complexes, but this feature had not yet been demonstrated in human disease until the work of the Kunkel laboratory. The Rockefeller University GCRC again provided the opportunity to validate and extend this observation [6]. A young man with lupus presented with an acute exacerbation characterized by high fever of 40° to 42°C, diffuse erythematosus rash involving the butterfly area of the face and other areas, acute arthritis, and increased proteinuria (Figure 20.1). This exacerbation occurred after he fell asleep under a sunlamp that he was using to obtain a healthy looking suntan during a dark and wintry New York season.

The practice in the Kunkel laboratory was to collect a serum sample at every clinic visit, and four samples of serum were available prior to the flare. We analyzed all sera extensively before and after the acute exacerbation time point (at the beginning of the third month in Figure 20.1). The four sera before the exacerbation all contained an

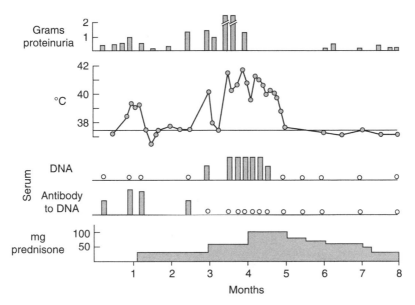

**FIGURE 20.1.** *This patient with lupus had a severe exacerbation after falling asleep under a sunlamp. This occurred at the end of the third month in this chart and was characterized by high fever, increased proteinuria, and widespread skin rash. Serum samples were available at four time points prior to the exacerbation and at many subsequent time points. Antibody to double-strand DNA was detectable in all the four sera prior to the exacerbation but replaced with detectable circulating DNA antigen and no detectable antibody in many samples during the period of high fever and increased proteinuria. These findings could be consistent with a period of antigen-antibody complex formation and antigen excess. (From J. Clin. Invest. 1966; 45: 1/32–1/40)*

antibody to DNA. The serum at the time of exacerbation and for 2 months following showed an absence of an antibody; instead, a DNA antigen was present. The patient was treated with large doses of prednisone, and ultimately, the fever subsided followed by decrease in proteinuria and disappearance of the DNA antigen. These data were compelling in suggesting that the acute exacerbation resulted from immune complexes of DNA and antibody to DNA. A year later, Kunkel and his associates showed that DNA-anti-DNA complexes could be eluted from lupus kidneys [7].

## 20.3 POWER OF THE IMMUNOFLUORESCENT ANTIBODY TECHNIQUE

One of the most important research tools in rheumatology to study autoantibodies is the immunofluorescent technique. In this technique, tissue sections or tissue culture cells are reacted with sera, and bound antibodies are detected with fluorescent-labeled antibody to the human immunoglobulin. In this way, autoantibodies that bind to different cellular antigens display distinct patterns of nuclear or cytoplasmic staining (except in situations when interference from multiple antibodies are present); the specificity of the antibody can be determined on the basis of the fluorescent pattern. Many autoantibodies in rheumatic diseases were initially observed with this method, followed by subsequent immunochemical and molecular studies to determine structural and functional identity.

An instructive example of the power of immunofluorescence was the first observation of the staining pattern of autoantibody to centromere proteins in the kinetochore region of the chromosome [8]. With a substrate of nonsynchronized Hep2 cells (containing cells in different phases of the cell cycle and some in mitosis), the staining pattern of this autoantibody displayed multiple dots in the nuclei. In a cell in mitosis (left frame, lower right), however, the dots were congregated at the mitotic plate (Figure 20.2). For several months, the cellular antigen remained a mystery in our laboratory; it was called the "Gildersleeve pattern." However, a unique observation central in our efforts to identify the antigen was the unusual pattern of antigens aligned with the condensed chromosomes during mitosis. Finally, we made a preparation of native condensed chromosomes (Fig. 20.2, right frame) and showed that the autoantibody reacted with the centromeric regions of chromosomes; this region is essential in cytokinesis or the segregation of condensed chromosomes in dividing daughter cells.

This autoantibody has been valuable to cell and molecular biologists studying mitotic division and was used to elucidate this cell process by immunoelectron microscopy [9]. In rheumatology, this autoantibody became a diagnostic biomarker for systemic sclerosis, and, in collaboration with Gerald Rodnan, an authority in scleroderma and head of the rheumatology division at the University of Pittsburgh, the antibody was shown to be associated with the CREST syndrome [10]. This

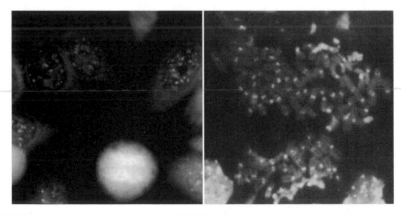

**FIGURE 20.2.** *The serum of a patient with CREST subset of scleroderma containing autoantibody to centromere proteins was examined with the immunofluorescent antibody technique, using non-synchronized Hep 2 cells as substrate (left frame). Characteristic staining pattern was fluorescence of dots in the nucleoplasm associated with dot-staining aligned at the mitotic plate in a cell undergoing mitosis (lower right region). The right frame shows immunofluorescent staining of a chromosome spread and dot staining restricted to the centromeric regions of the condensed chromosomes.*

autoantibody marker finally resolved a lively debate at that time as to whether an entity existed called the CREST syndrome.

## 20.4 PROFILES OF AUTOANTIBODIES AS DIAGNOSTIC BIOMARKERS

Certain autoantibodies show high specificity as disease biomarkers, and in this respect, anti-Sm stands as the prototype because it is present in SLE and rarely observed in other diseases. Anticentromere may be another such marker, especially for Raynaud's phenomenon, although this symptom can be idiopathic, lack disease association, or occur with CREST or systemic sclerosis. A finding that is not sufficiently emphasized is that profiles of autoantibodies are more important as diagnostic markers than individual autoantibodies. Anti-Sm, which is highly specific for SLE, is present in up to 15% to 20% of lupus patients, and therefore it is an antibody marker with high specificity but low sensitivity. The profile of autoantibodies for a particular disease may include several antibodies, some with high sensitivity and low specificity and others with low sensitivity but high specificity [11–13]. In addition, for each disease, the absence of antibodies of certain specificities is important in diagnostic profiling. For example, in mixed connective tissue disease, anti-U1 ribonucleoprotein (RNP) is an almost constant serological feature but, for this diagnosis, the antibody should occur in the absence of other autoantibodies. In contrast, anti-U1RNP is also present in lupus, but almost always other autoantibodies are present such as anti-Sm, anti-double-strand DNA, antihistones, or others.

## 20.5 TOWARD A BROADER APPRECIATION OF THE SIGNIFICANCE OF AUTOANTIBODIES

The conventional wisdom on autoantibodies is that they are nothing but bad news and can cause immune complex-mediated tissue inflammation. Although in rheumatology, serological testing is used in clinical practice, we have little, if any, understanding of why autoantibody responses to cellular protein antigens are initiated. However, some understanding of this autoimmune response is coming from cancer, where autoantibodies to oncogene products and to tumor suppressor proteins are being reported in increasing frequency [14]. Autoantibody responses to tumor-associated antigens (TAAs) can be stimulated by a variety of factors, including genetic mutations that produce altered proteins, overexpression of normal cellular proteins, aberrant expression of fetal proteins in malignant cells, ectopic localization of cellular proteins, and others. We have called autoantibodies to TAAs "reporters" from the immune system signaling incipient or ongoing malignant transformation [15]. In trying to understand the mechanisms for the autoantibody responses in rheumatic diseases like lupus and rheumatoid arthritis, we could benefit from the observations made in cancer immunology, which could be a goal of studies to come.

## ACKNOWLEDGMENT

The work summarized in this report has been supported by several grants from the National Institutes of Health, Bethesda, MD and by the W. M Keck Foundation of Los Angeles, CA.

## REFERENCES

1. Robbins WC, Holman HR, Deicher HR, et al. Complement fixation with cell nuclei and DNA in lupus erythematosus. Proc Soc Exp Biol Med 1957;96:575–579.

2. Seligman M. Mise en evidence dans le malades atteints de lupus erythemateux dissemine d'une substance determinant une reaction de precipitation avec l'acide desoxyribonuclei-que. CHR Acad Sci 1957;245:243–247.

3. Tan EM, Kunkel HG. Characteristics of a soluble nuclear antigen precipitating with sera of patients with systemic lupus erythematosus. J Immunol 1966;96:464–471.

4. Tsokos GC. In the beginning was Sm (Pillars of Immunology Series). J Immunol 2006;176:1295–1296.

5. Lerner MR, Steitz JA. Antibodies to small RNAs complexed with proteins are produced by patients with systemic lupus erythematosus. Proc Natl Acad Sci USA 1979;76:5495–5497.

6. Tan EM, Carr RI, Schur PH, et al. DNA and antibody to DNA in the serum of patients with systemic lupus erythematosus. J Clin Invest 1966;45:1732–1740.

7. Koffler D, Schur PH, Kunkel HG. Immunological studies concerning the nephritis of systemic lupus erythematosus. J Exp Med 1967;126:207–215.

8. Moroi Y, Peebles C, Fritzler MJ, Steigerwald J, Tan EM. Autoantibody to centromere (kinetochore) in scleroderma sera. Proc Natl Acad Sci 1980;77:1627–1631.

9. Brenner S, Pepper D, Berns MW, et al. Kinetochore structure, duplication and distribution in mammalian cells. Analysis by human autoantibodies from scleroderma patients. J Cell Biol 1981;91:95–102.

10. Tan EM, Rodnan G, Garcia I, et al. Diversity of antinuclear antibodies in progressive systemic sclerosis. Anti-centromere antibody and its relationship to CREST syndrome. Arthritis Rheum 1980;23:617–625.

11. Notman DD, Kurata N, Tan EM. Profiles of antinuclear antibodies if systemic rheumatic diseases. Ann Int Med 1975;83:464–469.

12. Tan EM. Immunospecificities of antinuclear antibodies. Arthritis Rheum 1977;20:187–181.

13. Nakamura RM, Tan EM. Recent progress in the study of autoantibodies to nuclear antigens. Human Pathol 1977;9:85–91.

14. Tan EM, Shi FD. Relative paradigms between autoantibodies in lupus and autoantibodies in cancer. Clin Exper Immunol 2003;134:169–177.

15. Tan EM, Zhang JY. Autoantibodies to tumor-associated antigens: Reporters from the immune system. Immunol Rev 2008;222:328–340.

# Chapter *21*

# *Cellular Regulation of Autoimmunity*

**Bevra H. Hahn, Ram Raj Singh, Ram Pyare Singh, Maida Wong, Brian Skaggs, Betty P. Tsao, and Antonio La Cava**

*UCLA School of Medicine, Rehabilitation Center, Los Angeles, CA*

## 21.1 OVERVIEW: THE PLAYERS IN INNATE AND ADAPTIVE IMMUNE RESPONSES

The immune system has multiple regulatory interactions that, in health, support a protective response against dangerous invaders from the outside world and attenuates that response when no longer needed and stores it in memory. When the balance between defense and regulation is imprecise, and/or when the stimuli are overwhelming, disease can result, such as uncontrolled infection, malignancies, and autoimmunity.

In the 75 years since the American College of Rheumatology was founded, many breakthroughs defining immune regulation have occurred. Although Edward Jenner tested vaccination with cowpox in 1796, it was in the 1900s that we learned that such protection resulted from antibodies, that antibodies were produced by plasma cells derived from B lymphocytes, and that B lymphocytes were stimulated to produce protective Immunoglobulin G(IgG) subsets of antibodies by help from T lymphocytes. A useful 2009 classification of protective and regulatory immune responses in terms of the innate and adaptive immune systems is presented in Figure 21.1.

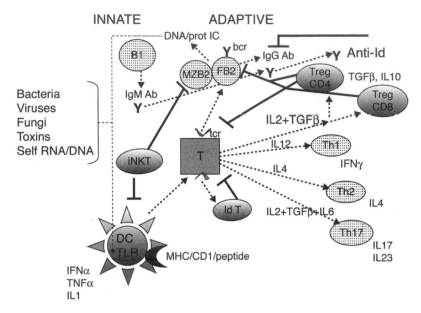

**FIGURE 21.1.** *Interplay of innate and adaptive immune systems in autoimmunity. The regulatory cells of the innate and adaptive systems are shown in shaded colors. The CD4+ and CD8+ Treg generated during immune responses, along with the DC educated to be "tolerant," interact to suppress B cells making autoantibodies and effector T cells helping that autoantibody production. Stippled cells are effects, which include B cells that make autoantibodies, as well as the Th1, Th2, and Th17 subsets of effector T cells (Teff). In the innate immune system, the invarant NKT (iNKT) cells interact with CD1 receptors on DC and B cells to suppress those targets when they are activated. Some of the cytokines known to be required to generate Treg and Teff, as well as major cytokines made by the effector cells, are also listed underneath each cell.*

Recently, it has become clear that these systems are linked in autoimmunity as well as in protective immunity.

Several cell types are specialized for the innate immune system, which are designed to eliminate danger quickly [1]. These cells recognize pathogen-associated molecular patterns (PAMPs), including those associated with bacteria, viruses, and fungi. Dendritic cells (of many types) and monocytes/macrophages are a first defense. Briefly, these cells search for foreign invaders, process the foreign proteins into antigens recognizable by T and B cells, and activate adaptive immune responses, as well as release microcidal mediators. Monocytes/macrophages are phagocytic and clear dangerous particles (e.g., immune complexes, apoptotic bodies, and oxidized lipids), bacteria, fungi, abnormal erythrocytes, lymphocytes, or platelets, and even small fibers. Another major innate immune cell is the neutrophil, which is characterized by phagocytosis and intracellular killing of bacteria. Natural killer lymphocytes (NK cells) are cytotoxic to virally infected cells. Innate-like B lymphocytes (marginal and B1 B cells) spontaneously and rapidly produce IgM natural antibodies (that recognize many microbial determinants) using primarily unmutated germline Ig genes. Innate-like T lymphocytes include gamma/delta and NK T cells, gamma/delta cells that respond to alkyl phosphate, and alkyl amines produced by bacteria; NK T cells probably recognize lipids from bacteria, which is presented in CD1d molecules.

## 21.2   LINKS BETWEEN INNATE AND ADAPTIVE IMMUNITY CAN PROMOTE AUTOIMMUNITY

An important clue to the origins of autoimmunity came with the observation that an IgM adaptive immune antibody to pneumococcus undergoing a single-point mutation acquired the ability to bind DNA [2]. A similar idea is that infection with the Ebstein-Barr virus (EBV), which is a possible trigger for systemic lupus erythematosus (SLE) and rheumatoid arthritis (RA), induces antibodies to an amino acid sequence also present in the self-antigen Sm B' [3]. Epitope spreading (a process in which T and B cells interact with increasing numbers of antigens as adaptive immune responses expand) allows anti-Sm responses to expand to antibodies against other U1 nuclear ribonucleoprotein (RNP) antigens, and eventually to nucleosome and DNA. Thus, a common viral infection in a genetically susceptible host could lead to SLE. Another innate/adaptive immunity link involves interactions between nucleic acids and toll-like receptors (TLRs) in DC and B cells. RNA from viruses or from RNA–protein in immune complexes can bind TLR7; CpG DNA from bacteria or DNA/protein immune complexes bind TLR9. Binding of TLR can activate DC and B cells, thus driving immune responses to self-antigens [4]. In general, when antibodies arise, T cells with T-cell receptors (TCRs) that can recognize processed antigens (either those that are bound by B-cell receptors or amino acid sequences within the receptors or their secreted Ig) also arise, and initial IgM responses can be switched to the more auto-pathogenic IgG [5].

## 21.3   INNATE AND ADAPTIVE REGULATORY NETWORKS FOR QUENCHING AUTOREACTIVITY

### 21.3.1   Idiotypic Networks

Ig antibody molecules and TCRs contain amino acid (AA) sequences (idiotypes [Ids]) that are antigenic, and induce anti-idiotypic responses. Some anti-Id antibodies and anti-Id T cells regulate cells that express the Id. Thus, anti-Ids can downregulate increased autoAb production; failure to do so is associated with disease flares in patients with SLE. In lupus-like disease of NZB/NZW F1 (BWF1) mice, the regulation of Id expression by administration of Ids or anti-Ids can modulate autoantibody production and nephritis, which indicates the importance of this type of immune regulation [6]. A small number of Ids found on Ig from many unrelated individuals, both murine and human, constitute a substantial proportion of the anti-DNA in tissue lesions of SLE, which include Ig deposited in skin lesions and in glomeruli. The same Ids are found on antibacterial Ig after infection and in healthy individuals. Thus, an Id/anti-Id regulatory pathway is a common mechanism based on recognition of aa sequences encoded by germline Ig genes widely available in the general population.

### 21.3.2 Regulatory CD4+ T Cells (CD4+ Treg)

At least two general types of Treg arise. The first type, which occurs in the thymus, is part of innate immunity and is not antigen specific. Innate Tregs and their role in suppressing autoimmunity were described in 1998 by Takahashi et al. [7]. These investigators showed that elimination of these cells in mice permitted development of organ-specific autoimmunity in some strains, and lupus-like systemic autoimmunity in others. Our laboratory has studied Treg induced in the adaptive immune system. For that purpose, we have administered to BWF1 mice an artificial 15-mer peptide (pConsensus; pCons) based on T-cell-activating AA sequences in the variable heavy chain (VH) regions of murine monoclonal anti-DNAs from BWF1 mice [8]. These cells differ from innate CD4+ Treg in that they are peptide-specific. Both types of CD4+ Treg are characterized by expression of CD4+ and CD25+, CTLA4, and GITR [9]. For suppressive function, Treg depend on upregulation of the transcription factor Foxp3 [10,11]. Interleukin-2 (IL-2) and transforming growth factor-beta (TGF-beta) are the major cytokines promoting development of CD4+ Treg, probably from CD4+CD25- T-cell precursors [12].

In our system, cells that are suppressed by CD4+ Treg include both CD4+CD25-helper/effector T cells and B2 cells, particularly those that make anti-DNA. In many and perhaps all systems, Tregs also exert their function by inducing a "tolerant" phenotype in the dendritic cells (DCs); the DC can then educate effector T cells to be tolerant rather than effectors [13]. CD4+ Treg suppress targets by contact; in our work, contact molecules on the Treg include membrane-bound LAP TGFb and GITR [9]. Patients with SLE have multiple defects in CD4+ Treg function; these include reduced quantities, reduced suppressive function (sometimes caused by glucocorticoid therapy), and impaired ability of target CD4+CD25- effector T cells to respond to Treg [14]. How the inability of human CD4+CD25- T-cells to respond to suppression by CD4+ Treg relates to the general abnormalities of T-cell activation characteristic of human SLE remains to be determined. Studies to induce Treg in these conditions, both by *ex vivo* education of T cells and by peptide immunization, are in progress. In this regard, we have shown that *in vitro* stimulation of peripheral blood mononuclear cells from patients with SLE with pCons results in substantial expansion of functional CD4+ Treg, primarily in patients with anti-DNA [15].

### 21.3.3 Regulatory CD8+ T Cells (CD8+ Treg)

An important discovery about the regulatory cell network concerns the presence of adaptive CD8+ Treg [16]. Such cells are not cytotoxic; they suppress CD4+CD25-effector T cells in part by secretion of IL-10 or TGF-beta. CD8+ Treg are induced in human transplantation immunity in response to alloantigen disparities; they also participate in allergy and cancer, as well as in autoimmunity [17]. It is likely that DC, CD4+ Treg, and CD8+ Treg educate each other to be tolerant, with CD4+ Treg and

CD8+ Treg inducing increase in immunoglobulin-like transcript-3(ILT-3) and decrease in CD80/86 in DCs. Such tolerized DCs support expansion of Treg rather than of Teffectors. Our laboratory has induced peptide-responsive CD8+ Treg in BWF1 mice by administration of pCons [18], or by immunization with DNA encoding an Ig construct that contains the AA sequence of pCons [19]. Like CD4+ Treg, CD8+ Treg require expression of Foxp3 for their activity. They are also relatively resistant to apoptosis, in part because of upregulation of Bcl2 [20], and they probably depend on a tightly regulated expression of surface PD-1 to deliver suppression [21,22]. In our system CD8+ Treg target both CD4+CD25-helper T cells and anti-DNA B cells, partly via secretion of TGF-beta. Of note, a single adaptive transfer of CD8+ Treg cells to BWF1 mice delays appearance of onset of autoimmunity significantly [18].

### 21.3.4 NKT Cells: Innate B-Cell–Innate T-Cell Axis in Regulation of Autoimmunity

Marginal zone B cells that rapidly respond to blood-borne antigens and activate naïve CD4+ T cells are enriched in self-reactive B cells. Such innate B cells express high levels of CD1d, an antigen presenting molecule that activates innate T cells called natural killer T (NKT) cells. NKT cells respond to lipid antigens and act rapidly. Our new data show that NKT cells impart homeostatic control of marginal zone B cell population, which regulates the response to blood-borne antigens and self-reactive B cells [23]. Consistently, deficiency of CD1d exacerbates autoimmune nephritis and dermatitis in mice [24,25] whereas treatment with CD1d-binding lipid antigens suppresses lupus dermatitis [26].

### 21.4 SUMMARY

Recent understanding of the interactions between the effector cells of autoimmunity (helper/effector T cells, B cells, and DCs) and "tolerized" DCs, innate and adaptive CD4+ Tregs, adaptive CD8+ Tregs, and innate NK T cells have expanded the potential of inducing targeted regulation of dangerous autoimmune responses. Current studies emphasize the molecular interactions that determine whether auto-reactivity or regulation dominate an immune response. The future holds exciting possibilities of highly targeted strategies to bend the response between the effector and suppressor for the purpose of controlling disorders that include cancer, allergies, transplantation rejection, and autoimmunity.

### REFERENCES

1. Porcelli SA. Innate immunity. In Kelley's Textbook of Rheumatology, (8th ed.). New York: Elsevier; 2009.
2. Davidson A, Shefner R, Livneh A, et al. The role of somatic mutation of immunoglobulin genes in autoimmunity. Annu Rev Immunol 1987:5:85–108.

3. Poole BD, Gross T, Maier S, et al. Lupus-like autoantibodies occur in rabbits and mice after immunization with EBNA-1 fragments. J Autoimmun 2008;31:362–371.

4. Marshak- Rothstein A. Toll-like receptors in systemic autoimmune disease. Nat Rev Immunol 2006;6:823–835.

5. Singh RR, Hahn BH. Reciprocal T-B determinant spreading develops spontaneously in murine lupus: implications for pathogenesis. Immunol Rev 1998;1643:201–208.

6. Hahn BH, Kalsi JK. Idiotypes and idiotypic regulation in SLE. In: Dubois Lupus Erythematosus. (Wallace D, Hahn B, eds). Philadelphia, Lippincott, Williams and Wilkens; PA: 2009.

7. Takahashi T, Kuniyasu Y, Toda M, et al. Immunologic self-tolerance maintained by CD25+ CD5+ naturally anergic and suppressive T cells: induction of autoimmune disease by breaking their anergic/suppressive state. Int Immunol 1998;10:1969–1980.

8. Hahn BH, Singh RR, Wong WK, et al. Treatment with a consensus peptide based on amino acid sequences in autoantibodies prevents T cell activation by autoantigens and delays disease onset in murine lupus. Arthritis Rheum 2001;44:432–441.

9. La Cava A, Ebling FM, Hahn BH. Ig-reactive CD4+ CD25+ T cells from tolerized (New Zealand Black x New Zealand White) F1 mice suppress in vitro production of antibodies to DNA. J Immunol 2004;173:3542–3548.

10. Sakaguchi S, Yamaguchi T, Nomura T, et al. Regulatory T cells and immune tolerance. Cell 2008;133:775–787.

11. La Cava A, Fang CJ, Singh RP, et al. Manipulation of immune regulation in systemic lupus erythematosus. Autoimmun Rev 2005;4:515–519.

12. Zheng SG, Wang J, Horwitz DA. Cutting edge: Foxp3+ CD4+ CD25+ regulatory T cells induced by IL-2 and TGF-beta are resistant to Th17 conversion by IL-6. J Immunol 2008;180:7112–7116.

13. Coquerelle C, Moser M. Are dendritic cells central to regulatory T cell function? Immunol Lett 2008;119:12–16.

14. Valencia X, Lipsky PE. CD4+ CD25+ Foxp3+ regulatory T cells in autoimmune diseases. Nat Clin Pract Rheumatol 2007;3:619–626.

15. Hahn BH, Anderson M, Le E, et al. Anti-DNA Ig peptides promote Treg cell activity in systemic lupus erythematosus patients. Arthritis Rheum 2008;58:2488–2497.

16. Skaggs BJ, Singh RP, Hahn BH. Induction of immune tolerance by activation of CD8(+) T suppressor/regulatory cells in lupus-prone mice. Hum Immunol 2008;69:790–796.

17. Vlad G, Cortesini R, Suciu- Foca N. CD8+ T suppressor cells and the ILT3 master switch. Hum Immunol 2008;69:681–686.

18. Hahn BH, Singh RP, La Cava A, et al. Tolerogenic treatment of lupus mice with consensus peptide induces Foxp3-expressing, apoptosis-resistant, TGFbeta-secreting CD8+ T cell suppressors. J Immunol 2005;175:7728–7737.

19. Ferrera F, La Cava A, Rizzi M, et al. Gene vaccination for the induction of immune tolerance. Ann NY Acad Sci 2007;1110:99–111.

20. Singh RP, La Cava A, Wong M, et al. CD8+ T cell mediated suppression of autoimmunity in a murine lupus model of peptide-induced immune tolerance depends on Foxp3 expression. J Immunol 2007;178:7649–7657.

21. Fife BT, Bluestone JA. Control of peripheral T-cell tolerance and autoimmunity via the CTLA-4 and PD-1 pathways. Immunol Rev 2008;224:166–182.

22. Singh RP, La Cava A, Hahn BH. Pconsensus peptide induces tolerogenic CD8+ T cells in lupus-prone (NZBxBZW)F1 mice by differentially regulating Foxp3 and PD1 molecules. J Immunol 2008;180:2069–2080.

23. Wen X, Yang J, Singh RR. iNKT cells regulate B cell development and homeostasis in the periphery. Exp Biol 2008:669:17.

24. Yang J-Q, Wen X, Liu H, et al. Examining the role of CD1d and natural killer T cells in the development of nephritis in a genetically lupus-susceptible model. Arthritis Rheum 2007:56:1219–1233.

25. Yang J, Chun T, Liu H, et al. CD1d-deficiency exacerbates inflammatory dermatitis in MRL-lpr/lpr mice. Eur J Immunol 2004:34:1723–1732.

26. Yang J, Saxena V, Xu H, et al. Repeated α-galactosylceramide administration results in expansion of NKT cells and alleviates inflammatory dermatitis in MRL-lpr/lpr mice. J Immunol 2003:171:4439–4446.

# Chapter 22

# Modern Biology/Bone and Cartilage Biology

**Steven R. Goldring and Mary B. Goldring**

*Hospital for Special Surgery, New York, NY*

## 22.1 BONE BIOLOGY

The discovery that the receptor activator of nuclear factor-kappa B (NF-kappa B) ligand (RANKL) and its receptor (RANK) are required for osteoclast differentiation and function initiated a new era in the field of bone cell biology [1–3]. Of note, RANKL was originally cloned and identified as tumor necrosis factor activation-induced cytokine (TRANCE), which is a T-cell–derived factors that regulates dendritic cell function [2,4]. This observation confirmed previous studies that established a link between immune and bone-cell regulation and helped to foster the development of the interdisciplinary field of osteoimmunology [5].

The role of RANKL in mediating bone destruction in an animal model of rheumatoid arthritis (RA) was initially reported by Kong et al. [6]. They showed that blocking the activity of RANKL by treating the arthritic animals with the soluble receptor osteoprotegerin (OPG) markedly attenuated the development of joint erosions. Subsequently, these observations were confirmed using genetic approaches and/or treatment with OPG in several different animal models [7–10]. These results provided convincing evidence that osteoclasts were required for pathologic bone loss in inflammatory arthritis and, importantly, that targeting RANKL was effective in

*The ACR at 75: A Diamond Jubilee*
Copyright © 2009 by John Wiley & Sons, Inc.

preventing osteoclast-mediated bone resorption. These initial studies in animal models led to the development of an alternate strategy for therapeutic targeting of RANKL using a humanized monoclonal antibody, and recent trials have confirmed the efficacy of RANKL blockade in the treatment of systemic osteoporosis, RA, and pathologic bone loss associated with bone metastases [11–14].

A hallmark of the articular bone lesion in RA is the virtual absence of bone repair, which is indicative of a dissociation between bone resorption and formation, which are tightly coupled under physiologic bone remodeling conditions [15]. Insights into the mechanism underlying the impaired bone formation associated with the marginal joint erosions was provided by a recent publication by Diarra et al. [16], who demonstrated that RA synovial fibroblasts produced an inhibitor of bone formation, Dickkopf-1 (DKK-1). DKK-1 is a member of a family of proteins that acts as inhibitors of the wingless (Wnt)-signaling pathway, which is involved in the regulation of multiple cellular activities, including bone formation and remodeling. The Wnts interact with two families of receptors, lipoprotein-related protein (LRP)5 or LRP6 and Frizzled (Fz). The importance of the constituents of this bipartite receptor complex in regulating bone loss was revealed by the observation that loss-of-function mutations in LRP5 are associated with the human disorder osteoporosis pseudoglioma syndrome, which is characterized by severely decreased bone mass. In contrast, gain-of-function mutations in LRP5 are associated with high bone mass [17–19]. Binding of the Wnt proteins to the receptor complex activates two pathways: the Beta-catenin canonical pathway and the $Ca^{2+}$ noncanonical pathway. Activation of the canonical pathway results in translocation of β-catenin to the nucleus where it interacts with T-cell factor (Tcf)/lymphoid enhancing factors (Lefs), which are transcription factors that control the expression of target genes that regulate osteoblast differentiation.

More evidence to implicate DKK-1 in impaired bone remodeling in RA was provided in the studies by Diarra et al. [16], who demonstrated that DKK-1 levels were elevated in the sera of patients with RA. They then employed *in vitro* cell cultures to show that tumor necrosis factor (TNF)-α increased DKK-1 levels in RA synovial fibroblasts, which links TNF-α to both inflammatory processes and suppression of bone formation and repair. They next showed that blockade of DKK-1 with a monoclonal antibody against DKK-1 partially restored bone repair in three different animal models of inflammatory arthritis. More importantly, they demonstrated that the treatment resulted in prevention of osteoclast-mediated bone resorption. These findings confirmed the work of other investigators, who showed that the increase in bone mass associated with activation of the Wnt signaling cascade was related not only to an increase in bone formation but also to an inhibition of bone resorption; this effect is mediated by downregulation of RANKL and induction of OPG.

Genetic analysis of humans with high bone mass phenotypes has led to the discovery of the Sost gene product sclerostin, which is an additional Wnt pathway inhibitor [20]. Van Buchem's disease and sclerosteosis are rare genetic disorders characterized by striking increases in bone mass. Genetic analysis has revealed that sclerosteosis results from loss of function of the Sost gene product and van Buchem's disease is associated with downregulation of the Sost gene related to partial deletion of the regulatory region [21,22]. Of note, osteocytes are the principle source of sclerostin [23]. These cells, which are embedded in the mineralized bone matrix and function as mechanosensors, regulate bone mass by modulating bone remodeling. Mechanical loading decreases osteocyte-derived sclerostin levels that result in upregulation of Wnt signaling and enhanced bone formation [24]. The past decade has witnessed the implementation of parathyroid hormone (PTH) into clinical practice as an anabolic agent to increase systemic bone mass is osteoporosis [25,26], and recent studies suggest that the modulation of osteocyte sclerostin may contribute to the anabolic effect of parathyroid hormone on bone [24,27]. In preliminary studies, neutralizing monoclonal antibodies to sclerostin have been shown to increase bone mass in a rat model of osteoporosis [28], which established the precedent for the development of additional therapeutic agents targeting the Wnt pathway in disorders associated with decreased bone mass.

In summary, the discovery of the RANKL/OPG system and identification of the essential role of the Wnt pathway in regulation of bone remodeling have created new opportunities for developing more effective approaches for treating disorders of bone remodeling. Advances also have been made in understanding the role of genetic factors that control bone mass and in defining the relationship between the skeletal system and other organ systems, which include the neural system and adipose tissue [29–32]. Algorithms for diagnosing disorders of bone remodeling employing biomarkers and additional patient-derived information also are being perfected, which permits improved detection of skeletal disorders and more effective assessment of therapeutic interventions [33].

## 22.2  CARTILAGE

Substantial advances have occurred in defining the cellular composition and structural organization of articular cartilage [34–36]. Chondrocytes from the superficial and deep zones demonstrate differences in the expression of molecules, which include lubricin that is localized to the superficial zone, where it plays an essential role in boundary mode lubrication. In addition, the expression of regulatory molecules such as parathyroid hormone related protein (PTHrP) by superficial zone chondrocytes, as well as Indian hedge hog (Ihh) and Runx2 by deep zone chondrocytes, may contribute to the zonal differences in matrix composition and function [37,38].

Chondrocytes exist at low oxygen tension, especially within the deep zones. *In vitro* studies suggest that they may adapt to this environment in part by upregulating hypoxia inducible factor-1α (HIF-1α). HIF-1α regulates several genes associated with cartilage anabolism and chondrocyte differentiation, which include vascular endothelial growth factor (VEGF) and Sox9 [39,40]. Hypoxia and other forms of stress regulate growth arrest and DNA damage (GADD) 45β, which was previously implicated as an antiapoptotic factor during genotoxic stress and cell cycle arrest in other cell types; in our studies, it seems to act as a survival factor in normal articular chondrocytes [41].

Recent studies have shown that aging is associated with alteration in the content, composition, and structural organization of collagen and proteoglycan [42,43].

These changes have been attributed to an overall decrease in chondrocyte anabolism and accumulation of advanced glycation end products (AGEs) that enhance collagen crosslinking [44]. The accumulation of cartilage matrix proteins modified by oxidative stress associated with the aging process may also contribute to diminished chondrocyte anabolic capacity and decreased cell survival [45].

Although the topographical distribution of synovial inflammation and cellular mechanisms of direct cartilage matrix destruction exhibit different patterns in RA and osteoarthritic (OA), both conditions are associated with deregulated chondrocyte anabolic and catabolic activities. In OA, injury to the cartilage matrix and/or adverse effects of mechanical loading in conjunction with genetic factors and aging play major contributory roles. In RA, the inflamed synovium is a major source of proinflammatory cytokines and cartilage matrix-degrading proteinases. Synovial inflammation also may be present in many patients with OA and could provide a source of cytokines and cartilage-degrading proteinases, although it seems that these degradative enzymes are primarily produced by chondrocytes [46,47].

Matrix metalloproteinases (MMPs), which include the collagenases (MMP-1, MMP-8, and MMP-13), the gelatinases (MMP-2 and MMP-9), stromelysin-1 (MMP-3), and membrane type I (MT1) MMP (MMP-14), have been implicated in cartilage collagen degradation in OA and RA [48]. Other MMPs and many members of the reprolysin-related proteinases of the ADAM (a disintegrin and metalloproteinase) family are expressed in cartilage. ADAMTS (ADAM with thrombospondin-1 domains) -4 and -5 are now regarded as the principal aggrecan-degrading enzymes in cartilage, and inhibitors have been developed for therapeutic intervention in OA [49,50].

*In vivo* and *in vitro* studies have shown that chondrocytes produce a broad spectrum of inflammatory mediators, cytokines such as interleukin-1β (IL-1β) and TNF-α, and chemokines that contribute by autocrine mechanisms to deregulated chondrocyte function [51–53]. IL-1β is a potent inducer of *COX2*, *MMP13*, and *NOS2* gene expression by chondrocytes. These effects are mediated by transcription factors, which include NF-κB, C/EBP, AP-1, and ETS family members [54,55]. IL-1β also uses these mechanisms to suppress the expression of many anabolic genes, including *COL2A1* and *CD-RAP*/MIA [56,57]. The toll-like receptor (TLR) superfamily of receptors has also been implicated in deregulated chondrocyte function. Human articular chondrocytes express TLR1, 2, and 4, and evidence suggests that cartilage matrix products can increase the production of MMPs, nitric oxide (NO), prostaglandin E (PGE), and VEGF via activation of TLR2. In addition, chondrocytes express integrins that serve as receptors for fibronectin (FN) and type II collagen fragments, and ligation of these receptors by matrix-derived ligands increases production of proteinases, cytokines, and chemokines by chondrocytes [58].

Candidate gene studies and genome-wide linkage analyses have revealed polymorphisms or mutations in genes encoding matrix and signaling molecules that may determine OA susceptibility [59,60]. Evidence suggests that during OA progression, chondrocytes may be induced to recapitulate a developmental molecular program, which includes chondrocyte hypertrophy [61,62]. This may be associated with upregulation of COL10A1, MMP-13, and Runx2 gene expression in the deep zone of OA cartilage accompanied by advancement of the tidemark.

The past decade has witnessed remarkable advances in defining the composition and structural organization of articular cartilage and in defining the molecular mechanisms regulating the anabolic and catabolic activities of chondrocytes. In the next decade, this information will be applied to the development of more effective therapies for improving the outcomes in patients with OA and inflammatory arthritis. In addition, advances in the development of biomarker assays that reflect quantitative and dynamic changes in the synthetic and degradation products of the cartilage matrix hold promise for early diagnosis and more accurate monitoring of the efficacy of disease-modifying therapies for patients with joint disease [63,64].

## REFERENCES

1. Lacey DL, Timms E, Tan HL, et al. Osteoprotegerin ligand is a cytokine that regulates osteoclast differentiation and activation. Cell 1998;93:165–176.

2. Wong BR, Josien R, Lee SY, et al. TRANCE (tumor necrosis factor [TNF]-related activation-induced cytokine), a new TNF family member predominantly expressed in T cells, is a dendritic cell-specific survival factor. J Exp Med 1997,186.2075–2080.

3. Yasuda H, Shima N, Nakagawa N, et al. Osteoclast differentiation factor is a ligand for osteoprotegerin/osteoclastogenesis-inhibitory factor and is identical to TRANCE/ RANKL. Proc Natl Acad Sci U S A 1998;95:3597–3602.

4. Anderson DM, Maraskovsky E, Billingsley WL, et al. A homologue of the TNF receptor and its ligand enhance T-cell growth and dendritic-cell function. Nature 1997;390:175–179.

5. Takayanagi H. Osteoimmunology: shared mechanisms and crosstalk between the immune and bone systems. Nat Rev Immunol 2007;7:292–304.

6. Kong YY, Feige U, Sarosi I, et al. Activated T cells regulate bone loss and joint destruction in adjuvant arthritis through osteoprotegerin ligand. Nature 1999;402:304–309.

7. Li P, Schwarz EM, O'Keefe RJ, et al. RANK signaling is not required for TNFalpha-mediated increase in CD11(hi) osteoclast precursors but is essential for mature osteoclast formation in TNFalpha-mediated inflammatory arthritis. J Bone Miner Res 2004;19:207–213.

8. Pettit AR, Ji H, von Stechow D, et al. TRANCE/RANKL knockout mice are protected from bone erosion in a serum transfer model of arthritis. Am J Pathol 2001;159:1689–1699.

9. Redlich K, Hayer S, Ricci R, et al. Osteoclasts are essential for TNF-alpha-mediated joint destruction. J Clin Invest 2002;110:1419–1427.

10. Romas E, Sims NA, Hards DK, et al. Osteoprotegerin reduces osteoclast numbers and prevents bone erosion in collagen-induced arthritis. Am J Pathol 2002;161: 1419–1427.

11. Bone HG, Bolognese MA, Yuen CK, et al. Effects of denosumab on bone mineral density and bone turnover in postmenopausal women. J Clin Endocrinol Metab 2008;93:2149–2157.

12. Brown JP, Prince RL, Deal C, et al. Comparison of the effect of denosumab and alendronate on BMD and biochemical markers of bone turnover in postmenopausal women with low bone mass: A randomized, blinded, phase 3 trial. J Bone Miner Res 2009;24:153–161.

13. Cohen SB, Dore RK, Lane NE, et al. Denosumab treatment effects on structural damage, bone mineral density, and bone turnover in rheumatoid arthritis: A twelve-month, multicenter, randomized, double-blind, placebo-controlled, phase II clinical trial. Arthritis Rheum 2008;58:1299–1309.

14. Ellis GK, Bone HG, Chlebowski R, et al. Randomized trial of denosumab in patients receiving adjuvant aromatase inhibitors for nonmetastatic breast cancer. J Clin Oncol 2008;26:4875–4882.

15. Goldring SR, Goldring MB. Eating bone or adding it: The Wnt pathway decides. Nat Med 2007;13:133–134.

16. Diarra D, Stolina M, Polzer K, et al. Dickkopf-1 is a master regulator of joint remodeling. Nat Med 2007;13:156–163.

17. Boyden LM, Mao J, Belsky J, et al. High bone density due to a mutation in LDL-receptor-related protein 5. N Engl J Med 2002;346:1513–1521.

18. Gong Y, Slee RB, Fukai N, et al. LDL receptor-related protein 5 (LRP5) affects bone accrual and eye development. Cell 2001;107:513–523.

19. Little RD, Carulli JP, Del Mastro RG, et al. A mutation in the LDL receptor-related protein 5 gene results in the autosomal dominant high-bone-mass trait. Am J Hum Genet 2002;70:11–19.

20. Baron R, Rawadi G. Targeting the Wnt/beta-catenin pathway to regulate bone formation in the adult skeleton. Endocrinology 2007;148:2635–2643.

21. Balemans W, Patel N, Ebeling M, et al. Identification of a 52 kb deletion downstream of the SOST gene in patients with van Buchem disease. J Med Genet 2002;39:91–97.

22. Staehling-Hampton K, Proll S, Paeper BW, et al. A 52-kb deletion in the SOST-MEOX1 intergenic region on 17q12-q21 is associated with van Buchem disease in the Dutch population. Am J Med Genet 2002;110:144–152.

23. Bonewald LF, Johnson ML. Osteocytes, mechanosensing and Wnt signaling. Bone 2008;42:606–615.

24. Robling AG, Niziolek PJ, Baldridge LA, et al. Mechanical stimulation of bone in vivo reduces osteocyte expression of Sost/sclerostin. J Biol Chem 2008;283:5866–5875.

25. Jilka RL. Molecular and cellular mechanisms of the anabolic effect of intermittent PTH. Bone 2007;40:1434–1446.

26. Potts JT, Gardella TJ. Progress, paradox, and potential: Parathyroid hormone research over five decades. Ann N Y Acad Sci 2007;1117:196–208.

27. Bellido T. Downregulation of SOST/sclerostin by PTH: A novel mechanism of hormonal control of bone formation mediated by osteocytes. J Musculoskelet Neuronal Interact 2006;6:358–359.

28. Li X, Ominsky MS, Niu QT, et al. Targeted deletion of the sclerostin gene in mice results in increased bone formation and bone strength. J Bone Miner Res 2008;23:860–869.

29. Hsu YH, Xu X, Terwedow HA, et al. Large-scale genome-wide linkage analysis for loci linked to BMD at different skeletal sites in extreme selected sibships. J Bone Miner Res 2007;22:184–194.

30. Karscnty G. Transcriptional control of skeletogenesis. Annu Rev Genomics Hum Genet 2008;9:183–196.

31. Lee NK, Karsenty G. Reciprocal regulation of bone and energy metabolism. Trends Endocrinol Metab 2008;19:161–166.

32. Takeda S, Karsenty G. Molecular bases of the sympathetic regulation of bone mass. Bone 2008;42:837–840.

33. Kanis JA, Johnell O, Oden A, Johansson H, McCloskey E. FRAX and the assessment of fracture probability in men and women from the UK. Osteoporos Int 2008;19:385–397.

34. Eyre DR, Weis MA, Wu JJ. Articular cartilage collagen: An irreplaceable framework? Eur Cell Mater 2006;12:57–63.

35. Goldring MB. Cartilage and chondrocytes. In: Kelley's Textbook of Rheumatology, (Firestein GS, Budd RC, McInnes IB, Sergent JS, Harris ED, Ruddy S, eds) (8th ed.) Philadelphia, PA: WB Saunders; 2008.

36. Poole AR. Cartilage in health and disease. In: Arthritis and Allied Conditions: A Textbook of Rheumatology, (15th ed) (Koopman WS, ed.). Philadelphia PA.: Lippincott, Williams, and Wilkins; 2005, pp. 223–269.

37. Chen X, Macica CM, Nasiri A, et al. Regulation of articular chondrocyte proliferation and differentiation by indian hedgehog and parathyroid hormone-related protein in mice. Arthritis Rheum 2008;58:3788–3797.

38. Cheng C, Conte E, Pleshko-Camacho N, et al. Differences in matrix accumulation and hypertrophy in superficial and deep zone chondrocytes are controlled by bone morphogenetic protein. Matrix Biol 2007;26:541–553.

39. Lin C, McGough R, Aswad B, et al. Hypoxia induces HIF-1alpha and VEGF expression in chondrosarcoma cells and chondrocytes. J Orthop Res 2004;22:1175–1181.

40. Robins JC, Akeno N, Mukherjee A, et al. Hypoxia induces chondrocyte-specific gene expression in mesenchymal cells in association with transcriptional activation of Sox9. Bone 2005;37:313–322.

41. Ijiri K, Zerbini LF, Peng H, et al. Differential expression of GADD45beta in normal and osteoarthritic cartilage: Potential role in homeostasis of articular chondrocytes. Arthritis Rheum 2008;58:2075–2087.

42. Aigner T, Haag J, Martin J, et al. Osteoarthritis: Aging of matrix and cells—going for a remedy. Curr Drug Targets 2007;8:325–331.

43. Loeser RF. Molecular mechanisms of cartilage destruction: mechanics, inflammatory mediators, and aging collide. Arthritis Rheum 2006;54:1357–1360.

44. Verzijl N, Bank RA, TeKoppele JM, et al. AGEing and osteoarthritis: A different perspective. Curr Opin Rheumatol 2003;15:616–622.

45. Yang L, Carlson SG, McBurney D, et al. Multiple signals induce endoplasmic reticulum stress in both primary and immortalized chondrocytes resulting in loss of differentiation, impaired cell growth, and apoptosis. J Biol Chem 2005;280:31156–31165.

46. Benito MJ, Veale DJ, FitzGerald O, et al. Synovial tissue inflammation in early and late osteoarthritis. Ann Rheum Dis 2005;64:1263–1267.

47. Scanzello CR, Plaas A, Crow MK, Innate immune system activation in osteoarthritis: Is osteoarthritis a chronic wound? Curr Opin Rheumatol 2008;20:565–572.

48. Murphy G, Nagase H. Reappraising metalloproteinases in rheumatoid arthritis and osteoarthritis: destruction or repair? Nat Clin Pract Rheumatol 2008;4:128–135.

49. Arner EC. Aggrecanase-mediated cartilage degradation. Curr Opin Pharmacol 2002;2:322–329.

50. Plaas A, Osborn B, Yoshihara Y, et al. Aggrecanolysis in human osteoarthritis: Confocal localization and biochemical characterization of ADAMTS5-hyaluronan complexes in articular cartilages. Osteoarthr Cartil 2007;15:719–734.

51. Goldring SR, Goldring MB. The role of cytokines in cartilage matrix degeneration in osteoarthritis. Clin Orthop 2004:(427 Suppl) S27–36.

52. Aigner T, Fundel K, Saas J, et al. Large-scale gene expression profiling reveals major pathogenetic pathways of cartilage degeneration in osteoarthritis. Arthritis Rheum 2006;54:3533–3544.

53. Sandell LJ, Xing X, Franz C, et al. Exuberant expression of chemokine genes by adult human articular chondrocytes in response to IL-1beta. Osteoarthr Cartil 2008;16:1560–1571.

54. Goldring MB, Goldring SR. Osteoarthritis. J Cell Physiol 2007;213:626–634.

55. Goldring MB, Sandell LJ. Transcriptional control of chondrocyte gene expression. In: OA, Inflammation and Degradation: A Continuum, (Buckwalter J, Lotz M, Stoltz JF, eds). Amsterdam; The Netherlands: IOS Press; 2007, p. 118–142.

56. Imamura T, Imamura C, Iwamoto Y, et al. Transcriptional co-activators CREB-binding protein/p300 increase chondrocyte Cd-rap gene expression by multiple mechanisms including sequestration of the repressor CCAAT/enhancer-binding protein. J Biol Chem 2005;280:16625–16634.

57. Peng H, Tan L, Osaki M, et al. ESE-1 is a potent repressor of type II collagen gene (COL2A1) transcription in human chondrocytes. J Cell Physiol 2008;215:562–573.

58. Pulai JI, Chen H, Im HJ, et al. NF-kappa B mediates the stimulation of cytokine and chemokine expression by human articular chondrocytes in response to fibronectin fragments. J Immunol 2005;174:5781–5788.

59. Loughlin J. Polymorphism in signal transduction is a major route through which osteoarthritis susceptibility is acting. Curr Opin Rheumatol 2005;17:629–633.

60. Valdes AM, Spector TD. The contribution of genes to osteoarthritis. Rheum Dis Clin North Am 2008;34:581–603.

61. Aigner T, Bartnik E, Sohler F, et al. Functional genomics of osteoarthritis: On the way to evaluate disease hypotheses. Clin Orthop Relat Res. 2004:S138–S143.

62. Drissi H, Zuscik M, Rosier R, et al. Transcriptional regulation of chondrocyte maturation: Potential involvement of transcription factors in OA pathogenesis. Mol Aspects Med 2005;26:169–179.

63. Dayer E, Dayer JM, Roux-Lombard P. Primer: The practical use of biological markers of rheumatic and systemic inflammatory diseases. Nat Clin Pract Rheumatol 2007;3:512–520.

64. Rousseau JC, Delmas PD. Biological markers in osteoarthritis. Nat Clin Pract Rheumatol 2007;3:346–356.

Chapter *23*

# Advances in Gout: A Brief Personal Perspective

**William N. Kelley**

*University of Pennsylvania School of Medicine, Rheumatology Division, Philadelphia, PA*

Early in my medical school experience (1959–1963), I became particularly interested in gout. It was a common disease, often seriously debilitating, whose pathogenesis made sense, a pathognomic diagnostic test existed, and a reasonably effective treatment was available. In addition, I was excited by the notion that the disease was essentially unique to the human race because almost all other mammals still had functional uricase and, hence, were protected from the accumulation of uric acid; this meant that no animal models existed, and studies of the disease had to be performed in human subjects. An investigator could not substitute an *Escherichia coli,* a Sprague Dawley rat, or even a nude mouse as an experimental subject and try to convince us that the research findings were relevant to our patients. Finally, it was the "Disease of Kings and the King of Diseases" with a fascinating history going back well before the masterful description of gout by Sydenham in 1683, which is based in part on 34 years of personal affliction. What was there not to like?

By the mid-1960s, voluminous and very impressive data were available on essentially every aspect of the disease [1]. The essential role of uric acid and of hyperuricemia in the causation of acute gouty arthritis, the gouty tophus, and uric acid kidney stones were generally worked out, although some details remained to be defined more accurately. It was apparent that the hyperuricemia could be caused by an

*The ACR at 75: A Diamond Jubilee*
Copyright © 2009 by John Wiley & Sons, Inc.

overproduction of uric acid, a defect in renal excretion, or a combination of both, but the nature of these lesions was totally unclear after exclusion of the well-established secondary causes of hyperuricemia. The acute attack could be effectively treated with nonsteroidal anti-inflammatory drugs (NSAIDs), and/or colchicine and chronic maintenance therapy with these agents was standard. An important advance in treatment had occurred with the development of uricosuric agents in the early 1950s. These drugs were effective in patients with good renal function, and it was clear that long-term reduction in the serum urate concentration would, over time, reduce the frequency of acute attacks and lead to the resolution of tophaceous deposits. Such impressive advances in our knowledge were often based on highly sophisticated studies in human subjects. Several of the most successful physician scientists in the field during this period, Jay Seegmiller and Jim Wyngaarden, were heroes of mine and were to later become important personal mentors.

As noted, it was well established by the mid-1960s that some portion of patients with gout exhibited an overproduction of uric acid. Over the subsequent years, several causes of this overproduction have been defined. The first enzymatic defect to be described in patients with primary gout was reported in 1967. While working at the National Institutes of Health (NIH) in the laboratory of Jay Seegmiller, we discovered that patients with the Lesch-Nyhan syndrome had a complete deficiency of the enzyme hypoxanthine phosphoribosyltransferase (HPRT) [2]. These patients had hyperuricemia and an overproduction of uric acid, but they also had a syndrome of self-mutilation, choreoathetosis, and mental retardation. Shortly after this discovery, we found a partial deficiency of the same enzyme in some patients with gout but without any of the devastating features of the Lesch-Nyhan syndrome [3]. By 1969, we reported 18 patients with gout caused by partial HPRT deficiency (now termed the Kelley-Seegmiller syndrome) from our analysis of gouty patients followed at the NIH [4]. Based on this population, we estimated that the incidence of this disorder could be as high as 5% of the gouty population; subsequent experience would suggest that it is less common than this, but no detailed analysis of its incidence has been conducted to our knowledge. Because the enzyme is encoded by DNA on the X chromosome, males are most severely affected. The females who are heterozygous for the mutated gene do have an accelerated rate of purine biosynthesis *de novo* and many become hyperuricemic after menopause; some will develop gout.

In 1972, Sperling et al. [5] described the first of several families with an elevated activity of phosphoribosylpyrophosphate (PRPP) synthetase as a cause of overproduction of uric acid in a gouty patient. Subsequent studies have confirmed that this disease, like the deficiency of HPRT, is X-linked. For both HPRT deficiency and PRPP synthetase overactivity, an elevated intracellular level of PRPP seems to be the basis of the increased uric acid production.

Only recently have we begun to understand the nature of the renal defects that seem to cause hyperuricemia in some and perhaps the majority of patients with gout. A polymorphism in the SLC2A9 gene was identified with hyperuricemia and gout in several genome-wide association studies [6–10]. In a more recent study of more than 33,000 participants by Fox and co-workers [11], two additional genes associated with renal urate transport and expressed on the apical membrane of renal proximal tubule cells (ABCG2, SLC17A3) were found to have missense mutations that were associated with an increased risk of hyperuricemia and gout. They also confirmed the earlier finding of gout associated with the polymorphism in the SLC2A9 gene as described above. The presence of all six risk alleles was associated with up to a 40-fold risk of developing gout.

These latter studies required large populations of people assembled over many years in multiple cohorts on two continents as well as a small village of talented scientists in the fields of epidemiology, medical informatics, genomics, and clinical medicine. We may well learn about additional polymorphisms tied to hyperuricemia and gout from these investigators. Finally, the possibility exists that a better understanding of other features of the metabolic syndrome, of which hyperuricemia is a part, will come from these important discoveries.

In my opinion, the most important advance in the treatment of hyperuricemia in the last 50 years was the development of allopurinol, a potent inhibitor of xanthine oxidase. The drug was developed by Trudy Elion and George Hitchings in the Wellcome Research Laboratories in 1963, where the early purine analogs used for cancer chemotherapy, 6-mercaptopurine, and immunosuppression, azathioprine, were also discovered. For these discoveries, they shared the Nobel Prize in Medicine in 1988.

The early clinical studies showing the effectiveness of this agent in blocking uric acid synthesis were carried out at Duke University [12,13]. Although allopurinol proved to have serious side-effects in a small number of patients, particularly when the standard dose was not reduced in the presence of renal insufficiency, in general, it was found to be highly effective and well tolerated. Despite early concerns about off-target effects of the drug, which turned out to be of little, if any, consequence, the drug became a mainstay for virtually every patient with gout. Indeed, over these many decades, allopurinol has been widely used and the vast majority of gouty patients have been well controlled. It is perhaps of more than passing interest that it was the last drug approved for the treatment of hyperuricemia, now over 40 years ago. For most patients, one can assure them that over time and with full compliance, this treatment will prove to be highly effective in controlling their illness.

From my personal perspective, I believe the success of allopurinol in patients with gout had an unintended consequence on research in the field. Patients who were formerly treated by subspecialists could be handled by generalists, and over the years, this represented about 90% of the gouty population. The corollary to this is that far fewer gouty patients were referred to the large academic centers. Fellows, residents, and medical students were no longer exposed to or challenged by this large and interesting group of patients. Faculty conceived that the problems remaining to be solved with the gouty population were no longer a priority because treatment was so effective. Perhaps making matters worse from this perspective, even the common question posed concerning when to treat asymptomatic hyperuricemia was no longer asked when uric acid was removed from routine laboratory testing panels sometime in the 1990s.

In my own laboratory, we continued to pursue the control of human purine metabolism, as well as the characteristics of the human HPRT protein and gene, including the specific nature of the many mutations that cause the enzyme deficiency. However, much of our focus shifted to other diseases of the purine pathway of more scientific relevance and interest, such as the deficiencies of adenosine deaminase, purine nucleoside phosphorylase, and adenine phosphoribosyltransferase, none of which were relevant to gout.

We also began to consider the possibility that gene therapy could be used to treat patients with the Lesch-Nyhan syndrome; in this disease, the hyperuricemia could be very effectively managed with allopurinol, but it had no effect on improving their devastating neurologic disease. Based on this shift in direction, we developed a new technique to conduct gene therapy in experimental animal models using modified DNA viruses as vectors to carry the gene of interest directly into the appropriate cells, tissues, or organs [14]. This form of gene therapy, which now termed *in vivo* gene therapy, as contrasted to *ex vivo* approaches used prior to our work, is the approach generally being tested today, but again it is not relevant to gout.

Many of our trainees moved into other areas of purine metabolism where their contributions could be important but are not relevant to gout. Although many examples could be cited, perhaps the most interesting is the work from Ed Holmes' laboratory. He and his coworkers did the pioneering work, and they demonstrated the possibility that aminoimidazole carboxamide riboside (AICAR) had a beneficial effect in ischemic muscle and that AICAR might be useful as a therapeutic agent [15,16]. Others have now demonstrated that AICAR can induce a phenotype characteristic of conditioned skeletal muscle in the absence of exercise [17]; some have suggested this effect may be a future exercise in a pill.

Finally, I want to say a few words about my wonderful experiences with rheumatology and the American College of Rheumatology (ACR). Early in my career, I had the opportunity to work closely with Ted Harris, Shaun Ruddy, and Clem Sledge and to participate in the creation of a new textbook in rheumatology. At the time we began, I was also Chief of the Division of Rheumatology at Duke. So, even though I strayed a bit from the field as I moved to other leadership positions in Ann Arbor, MI, and Philadelphia, PA, I stayed close to the specialty and to the ACR (or the American Rheumatism Association [ARA], as it was called then). Hence, I had the great pleasure of working with many outstanding colleagues and of serving in many different roles with the ACR, including a year as President in the mid-1980s. I also was blessed and deeply appreciative of recognition by the membership of the ACR with both the Presidential Gold Medal award and the Masters designation. As others will no doubt summarize elsewhere in this volume, the trek from the beginnings of the ARA to the current premier status of the ACR as a global leader of medical specialty societies has been tortuous. To the extent I was helpful along the way, I was deeply appreciative of the opportunity.

## REFERENCES

1. Wyngaarden JB, Kelley WN. Gout and Hyperuricemia. New York: Grune and Stratton; 1976.

2. Seegmiller JE, Rosenbloom FM, Kelley WN. Enzyme defect associated with a sex-linked human neurological disorder and excessive purine synthesis. Science 1967;155:1682–1684.

3. Kelley WN, Rosenbloom FM, Henderson JF, et al. A specific enzyme defect in gout associated with overproduction of uric acid. PNAS 1967;57:1735–1739.

4. Kelley WN, Greene ML, Rosenbloom FM, et al. Hypoxanthine-guanine phosphoribosyl-transferase deficiency in gout. Ann Int Med 1969;70:155–206.

5. Sperling O, Eilam G, Persky-Brosh S, et al. Accelerated erythrocyte 5-phosphoribosyl-1-pyrophosphate synthesis. A familial abnormality associated with excessive uric acid production and gout. Biochem Med 1972;6:310–316.

6. Li S, Sanna S, Maschio A, et al. The *GLUT9* gene is associated with serum uric acid levels in Sardinia and Chianti cohorts. PLoS Genet 2007;3:e194.

7. Wallace C, Newhouse SJ, Braund P, et al. Genome-wide association study identifies genes for biomarkers of cardiovascular disease: serum urate and dyslipidemia. Am J Hum Genet 2008;82:139–149.

8. Doring A, Gieger C, Mehta D, et al. SLC2A9 influences uric acid concentrations with pronounced sex-specific effects. Nat Genet 2008;40:430–436.

9. Vitart V, Rudan I, Hayward C, et al. SLC2A9 is a newly identified urate transporter influencing serum urate concentration, urate excretion and gout. Nat Genet 2008;40:437–442.

10. Stark K, Reinhard W, Neureuther K, et al. Association of common polymorphisms in *GLUT9* gene with gout but not with coronary artery disease in a large case-control study. PLoS ONE 2008;3:e1948.

11. Dehghan A, Kottgen A, Yang Q, et al. Association of three genetic loci with uric acid concentration and risk of gout: a genome-wide association study. Lancet 2008;372:1953–1961.

12. Rundles RW, Wyngaarden JB, Hitchings GH, et al. Effects of a xanthine oxidase inhibitor on thiopurine metabolism, hyperuricemia and gout. Trans Assoc Amer Phys 1963;76:126.

13. Wyngaarden JB, Rundles RW, Silberman HR, et al. Control of hyperuricemia with hydroxypyrazolopyrimidine, a purine analogue, which inhibits uric acid synthesis. Arth Rheum 1963;6:306.

14. U.S. Patent 5,672,344. Viral-Mediated Gene Transfer System. Inventors: William N Kelley, Thomas D Palella, Myron Levine. 1997.

15. Swain JL, Hines JJ, Sabina RL, et al. Accelerated repletion of ATP and GTP pools in postischemic canine myocardium using a precursor of purine de novo synthesis. Circ Res 1982;51:102–105.

16. Sabina RL, Patterson D, Holmes EW. 5-amino-4-imidazolecarboxamide riboside (Z-riboside) metabolism in eukaryotic cells. J Biol Chem 1985;260:6107–6114.

17. Narkar VA, Downes M, Yu RT, et al. AMPK and PPARδ agonists are exercise mimetics. Cell 2008;134:405–415.

# Chapter 24

# Gout and the Other Crystal-Associated Diseases

**H. Ralph Schumacher, Jr.**

*VA Medical Center, Philadelphia, PA*

Gout has been recognized since antiquity, and it was one of the four types of arthritis in a list at the time of the American Revolution. At this 75th anniversary of what is now the American College of Rheumatology (ACR), founded in 1934 when I was 1 year old, the management, differential diagnosis, and study of gout has attracted an impressive list of America's leading rheumatologists who have made an ongoing series of important advances.

A 1935 second edition of a rheumatology textbook by Ralph Pemberton [1] had only the following to say about gout in a 432-page book:

> **Gout or Gouty Arthritis**, - While gout no longer occupies the position it apparently once held, at least in so far as the number of papers in the current literature on this topic are an index, it does, however, according to Hench, occur more frequently than is generally recognized and it still presents the classical clinical picture. Part of the failure to recognize the disease is perhaps due to the fact that some cases are included under the diagnosis of either atrophic or hypertrophic arthritis.

*The ACR at 75: A Diamond Jubilee*
Copyright © 2009 by John Wiley & Sons, Inc.

Although gout is clinically separable from arthritis, Knaggs believes that it has a definite pathogenetic relationship, in that joint lesions probably precede the deposition of sodium-rate. (presumably he meant urate) These deposits characterize gout and lead to further mechanical damage to the joint structures.

It is often said that research and training about gout and other crystal-associated diseases have been neglected over the years. This situation is in part because we have had no new therapies since about 1963 until very recently. Furthermore, many training programs have focused more on the well-funded, rapidly evolving area of immunology. Nevertheless, a continuing flow of work is available, and researchers deserve recognition.

Probenecid, a uricosuric, which was the first drug established as a urate-lowering agent for gout, was identified during studies for methods to inhibit renal clearance and increase effectiveness of the recently discovered antibiotic, penicillin. John Talbott, Tsai Fan Yu, and Alexander Gutman used probenecid and were the leading investigators and teachers on gout during the 1950s. At that time, treatment of acute gout most often was with colchicine dosed until diarrhea, and interestingly, either hot or cold applications. Only recently were better-tolerated colchicine regimens shown and the effect of cold (but not heat) confirmed.

My first scientific paper and first presentation at the American Rheumatism Association (ARA) meeting in Atlantic City in 1963 before about 300 rheumatologists should have warned me that crystal-associated diseases would play an important part in my career. I reported that arthropathy was a previously unrecognized feature of patients with hemochromatosis observed at University of California at Los Angeles (UCLA) and the Wadsworth VA Hospital and described (without explanation) in my paper that calcification was noted in a knee meniscus.

Zitnan and Sitaj had described patients with similar radiographic evidence of chondrocalcinosis in 1957 at a conference in France and in 1958 in a Czech journal. In 1961, Daniel McCarty et al. [2] first at Penn and later at Hahneman in Philadelphia, had rediscovered and taught about monosodium urate (MSU) crystals in joint fluid and then described what became known as calcium pyrophosphate dihydrate (CPPD) crystals in synovial fluids from similar patients in 1962 [2]. McCarty presented a follow up at the same 1963 ACR meeting. Although I had not seen inflammation or crystals in these first few patients with hemochromatosis arthropathy it eventually became clear to me and others that this disease was associated with CPPD deposition.

Although it was widely recognized in the 1940s [3] that urates could be observed deposited in joint cartilage, synovium, and bone, the 1953 monograph by Ropes and Bauer on synovial fluid described inflammation but no identification of crystals in gouty joint fluids. It was not until McCarty and Joe Hollander made the examination of joint fluid for crystals an essential part of clinical evaluation that several generations of investigators were stimulated to keep up studies on crystals. I had been doing a fellowship in Boston learning cell biology and electron microscopy (EM) to begin my studies on early synovitis. When I got my first job at Penn with Jim Wyngaarden (later director at National Institutes of Health) and Hollander, a persuasive young colleague, Paulding Phelps, drew me into using the EM and my laboratory to also study crystal-induced inflammation.

In 1963, Wayne Rundles at Duke reported a clinical trial of allopurinol, which revolutionized urate-lowering therapy. Allopurinol had been developed initially to prolong the half-life of 6-mercaptopurine (6-MP). In the late 1960s, gout and hyperuricemia received more attention with the beginning of studies identifying the Lesch Nyhan syndrome and the work by Bill Kelley, Jay Seegmiller, et al. identifying the deficiency of hypoxanthine guanine phosphoribosyltransferase (HGPRTase) and then Michael Becker's identification of increased phosphoribosylpyrophosphate (PRPP) synthetase as another cause of overproduction of uric acid.

By the 50th anniversary meeting of the ARA in Minneapolis in 1984, there were 11 papers on gout and a growing list of other crystal-associated diseases. One paper by Woolf et al. from the United Kingdom reported high levels of interleukin 1 (IL-1) in gouty synovial fluid, presaging our current interest in the inflammasome and IL-1. MSU crystals have now been shown to activate the NALP3 inflammasome with production of IL-1beta as part of their mechanism causing inflammation. Uric acid has also been identified as a likely adjuvant in immune reactions. Mechanisms for the spontaneous resolution of attacks have been investigated.

Observations on other crystals of importance (pathogenic or artefactual) in analyzing joint fluid such as apatite (basic calcium phosphate), oxalate, cholesterol, depot corticosteroids, lipid liquid crystals, and cryoglobulins have come over the last 40 years largely in the United States. CPPD and apatite crystals, which have been extensively studied by Cheung and colleagues, not only can be associated with acute inflammation but also stimulate mitogenesis and metalloprotease synthesis in synovial and cartilage cells that may contribute to joint damage in osteoarthritis. Unfortunately, we have no measures to deplete these calcium crystals, which leaves a major area in need of research. Phosphocitrate is one molecule under investigation.

Ongoing activities include major efforts with Outcome Measures in Rheumatoid Arthritis (OMERACT) clinical trials to validate outcomes to give uniformity to clinical trials in gout; an ACR-European League Against Rheumatism (EULAR) joint project has been funded to reach consensus on what is a "gout flare," because reduction in flares along with resolution of tophi and improved function are key clinical outcomes that are needed to establish value to aggressive measures to normalize serum urate levels. Genetic studies are addressing genes involved in urate excretion and offer the possibility for more efficient blocking of sites such as URAT1 and creating better uricosurics.

The evolving studies on the connections between uric acid (soluble or crystals), cardiovascular risk, renal disease, hypertension, and metabolic syndrome will continue to demand attention and possibly lead to treatment recommendations.

Needs in this area include major educational efforts about gout because the diagnosis and treatment of this disease are still not ideal for many patients observed by primary care providers. Current drugs may not be used optimally. One small study from Taiwan suggested that HLA-B5801 may predict risk of allopurinol hypersensitivity, and if confirmed in Americans, it could alleviate some anxiety about our use of this drug. New agents, which are now specifically targeted for gout, including a totally different xanthine oxidase inhibitor, febuxostat, and pegylated uricase are under investigation, with each offering possibilities for the neglected patients with allopurinol hypersensitivity. These potent new agents increase the risk for gouty flares that occur with abrupt lowering of serum urate. Thus, better anti-inflammatory prophylaxis is needed and may involve agents directed at various chemokines and cytokines, including IL-1.

A series of books about gout and the other crystals have been published to update the status of the growing knowledge about crystals with examples from 1976 to 2006 [4,5]. These show the changing areas of emphasis and how each step of the investigation builds on earlier steps.

Studies and progress on gout have always had important international input. Many visiting researchers have presented important work at ACR meetings. At this 75th anniversary, I choose to focus mostly on our American contributions. At the risk of making some terrible omission, I close this review with a list of many American, Mexican, and Canadian ACR members who I have learned from and/or worked with and have contributed and continue to contribute to this field: Steve Abramson, Carlos Agudelo, Daniel Baker, Gene Ball, Michael Becker, Tom Benedek, Lan Chen, Herman Cheung, Hyon Choi, Bruce Cronstein, John Decker, Herb Diamond, Howard Duncan, Larry Edwards, Adel Fam, Jeffrey Fessel, Irving Fox, Alexander Gutman, Arthur Hall, Paul Halverson, Andy Healey, Michael Hershfield, Marc Hochberg, Joe Hollander, David Howell, Rick Johnson, Bill Kelley, Jim Klinenberg, Steve Malawista, Brian Mandel, Bill Martel, Dan McCarty, Ted Mikuls, Rollie Moskowitz, Tom Palella, Paulding Phelps, Ken Pritzker, Antonio Reginato, Gerry Rodnan, Ann Rosenthal, Larry Ryan, Ken Saag, Naomi Schlesinger, Jay Seegmiller, Peter Simkin, Jas Singh, Charley Smyth, Lief Sorensen, Isaias Spilberg, John Sundy, John Talbott, Bob Terkeltaub, Janitzia Vazquez-Mellado, Stan Wallace, Gerry Weissmann, Charlene Williams, Bob Wortmann, Jim Wyngaarden, and Tsai-fan Yü.

Interestingly, 10 gout and crystal experts, John Decker, Joe Hollander, Bill Kelley, Jim Klinenberg, Steve Malawista, Dan McCarty, Paulding Phelps, Gerry Rodnan, Charley Smyth, and Gerry Weissman have been among the presidents of the ACR (ARA).

## REFERENCES

1. Pemberton R. Arthritis and rheumatoid conditions. Their nature and treatment, (2nd ed.). Philadelphia, PA: Lea and Febiger; 1935, p. 432.

2. McCarty J, Kohn NN, Faires JS. The significance of calcium phosphate crystals in the synovial fluid of arthritic patients: the "pseudogout" syndrome. I. Clinical aspects. Ann Int Med 1962;56:711–737.

3. Bennett GA. The Joints. In: Pathology. (Anderson WAD, ed.) St. Louis MO, CV Mosly Co; 1948; p. 1330.

4. Talbott JH, Yü T-F. Gout and uric acid metabolism. New York: Stratton Intercontinental; 1976; p. 303.

5. Wortman RL, Schumacher HR, Becker MA, Ryan LM. (eds.). Crystal-Induced Arthropathies. New York, Taylor & Francis; 2006; p. 4427.

# Chapter 25

# Clinical Trials in Rheumatology: The Past 75 Years and a Glimpse into the Future

David T. Felson

*Boston University School of Medicine, Clinical/Research Training Unit, Boston, MA*

The past 75 years have experienced the emergence of highly effective treatments for many major rheumatic diseases. What once were a group of disabling illnesses characterized by physical disability have, with new treatments, become mostly controllable illnesses allowing affected patients to experience life's joys and live productive lives. This triumph of rheumatology treatment is in part caused by the development of randomized clinical trials, which permit rheumatologists to identify treatments that work. In the last 20 years, standardization and refinement of trial methodology has allowed greater distinction of more from less effective therapies and consequently led to improved effectiveness of treatments for patients.

Although natural history studies of persons receiving promising therapies can provide valuable information about the effectiveness of these therapies, this information is flawed by the tendency of rheumatic disease activity to wax and wane

*The ACR at 75: A Diamond Jubilee*
Copyright © 2009 by John Wiley & Sons, Inc.

(e.g., improvement for the patient on a novel treatment may be the natural waning of a flare of disease). Also, symptoms of rheumatic disease are often so subjective that a patient receiving a new therapy may perceive improvement and interpret that as evidence of treatment efficacy. It is only by testing treatments against others or against placebo in a randomized trial that definitive evidence on the efficacy of treatment is collected. Randomization, if effective, produces two groups that are equally likely to improve and where the only difference between them is the new therapy administered to one of the groups. If both groups are tracked carefully to the end of the study with all randomized patients evaluated, then the effect of the new treatment versus the control treatment can be assessed, and treatment efficacy can be determined.

In rheumatology, randomized trials were first undertaken almost 70 years ago in England by the Empire Rheumatism Council, which, for rheumatoid arthritis, tested the efficacy of aspirin, corticosteroids, gold, and hydroxychloroquine. Rheumatologists in the United States, with NIH support, developed the Cooperative Systematic Studies of Rheumatic Disease (CSSRD, also called the Cooperating Clinics) to conduct large multicenter trials of treatments for rheumatic diseases. All major second line drugs in rheumatoid arthritis prior to the introduction of biologics agents were evaluated by the CSSRD or the Empire Rheumatism Council.

## 25.1 SPECIFIC EXAMPLES OF TRIALS THAT CHANGED PRACTICE

In rheumatology, as in other fields, clinical trial evidence has sometimes served to disprove the efficacy of widely used treatments. Examples include trials showing that routine bed rest for back pain was no more effective than allowing patients ad-lib activity [1], as well as trials showing that penicillamine was ineffective for scleroderma [2]. Other trials producing essentially negative results have shown that steroid injections in regional soft tissue rheumatism are of marginal efficacy compared with injections of saline and that arthroscopy is ineffective as a treatment for knee osteoarthritis [3].

Even though trials showing that accepted treatments actually do not work are extraordinarily valuable, trials perhaps have their greatest effect when they either demonstrate the efficacy of a new therapy [e.g., tumor necrosis factor (TNF) inhibitor trials in rheumatoid arthritis) or when they test out a new conceptual approach to treatment [4]. The best example of the latter group of trials are those that evaluate aggressive early therapy of rheumatoid arthritis as a way of inducing remission in disease and preventing long-term structural damage. One common theme emerging from trials over the last 20 years is that existing treatment regimens for rheumatoid arthritis (e.g., pyramid approach with gradual introduction of disease-modifying antirheumatic drugs (DMARDs) and use of single agents) were not aggressive enough. This demonstration of improved outcomes was abetted in part by the careful development of trial outcome assessments, which showed that patients can continue to have active and disabling disease when treated with single conventional agents.

## 25.2   TRENDS IN TRIALS OVER THE LAST 20 YEARS

In the last 20 years, rheumatology trials have become increasingly numerous and also increasingly sponsored and performed by industrial sponsors [5] with a critical oversight function performed by the U.S. Food and Drug Administration (FDA) and European regulatory agencies. Many advances in trial design and methods have been spurred by FDA insistence on high-quality trials.

Among the important advances of the last 20 years has been the standardization of outcome measures. For many years, trial design in rheumatology was characterized by outcome measures that varied from trial to trial. Some outcome measures used were unlikely to change even with effective treatment (e.g., rheumatoid factor levels). In other circumstances, so many measures were assessed that one or more of them would show efficacy for a treatment by chance given the number of statistical tests performed. One major advance in the 1990s was the development and widespread acceptance of a core set of outcome measures for the evaluation of treatments in rheumatoid arthritis trials [6]. This core set consists of seven unique outcome measures that range from examination measures such as joint counts to patient measures such as pain and global assessments to a laboratory test (e.g., an acute phase reactant). This core set facilitated the development of composite measures of outcome, such as the American College of Rheumatology (ACR) definition of improvement [7] and the Disease Activity Score (DAS), and it spurred the creation of core sets in most other rheumatic diseases. This standardization and uniformity of trials in rheumatoid arthritis facilitated the development of new treatments. With these improved measures, response rates to new treatments could be compared with those of conventional therapy, and trials could be conducted with fewer patients.

In 2005, editors of medical journals required that trials undertaken be registered with the appropriate national trial registries. This system will ultimately serve as a mechanism to identify trials that were completed but whose results were not published, which will overcome some elements of publication bias.

## 25.3   NEW CHALLENGES FOR RHEUMATOLOGY TRIALS

The challenges for clinical trials over the next 10–20 years are new ones. First, rheumatology patients would be best served by the release of information from all trials undertaken, which includes those that suggest a treatment does not work. Publication bias concerning trials in rheumatology can result from the failure of small null trials to get published, which thereby limits accurate assessment of the efficacy of treatment. Trial registration will minimize publication bias but will not eliminate it. Second, whereas rheumatology trials, often with the urging of regulatory agencies, have sample sizes large enough to test treatment efficacy, recent evaluations of lupus trials and of trials in other areas of rheumatic disease suggest that many trials remain too small to be likely to detect the efficacy of treatments [8] Third, although many rheumatic disease patients are elderly, many trials exclude or under-represent such patients in part because of their high rate of comorbidity. Older subjects and those who are likely to be more representative of patients in the community need to be better represented in trials.

Ultimately, in many rheumatic diseases but especially in rheumatoid arthritis, a group of effective medications is available but there is little evidence as to how they compare. Treatment efficacy and safety need to be compared, but it may not be in the best interests of particular companies to carry out comparative studies nor is the FDA interested in such studies. Because some new treatments may not offer more efficacy but rather better safety than older ones, equivalence trials will be needed, which are trials that test whether a new drug is roughly equivalent in efficacy to an already available one. Such trials have become increasingly popular in other medical fields where multiple treatments are available such as in cardiology; in rheumatology, these trials are needed to define the rank order and unique usefulness of each treatment. Also, because of concerns about misrepresentation of trial results in trial reports, journal editors are already demanding and will increasingly require trial data to be made available to coauthors and statisticians who represent the journals and perhaps even to readers. This can permit a reanalysis of trial data to determine whether reported results are accurate.

Ultimately, the average response on treatment is reported but is not necessarily a valuable predictor of an individual's likely expected benefit or harm. First, although everyone may experience some benefit from a drug, the absolute benefit is not the same from person to person. In those who can expect only mild improvement either because of mild disease or genetic predisposition to drug response, a treatment's benefit may not outweigh its risks. However, for patients with greater expected absolute improvement, treatment will be indicated because efficacy benefits will outweigh potential risks.

Because of individual variations in drug metabolism and pharmacodynamics, treatment will increasingly become individualized. In certain patients, drug metabolism will be slow, which leads to higher levels of drug. In others, the opposite will occur and they may not respond to a given treatment. Mechanisms of disease are determined in large part by genetic differences from person to person and constitute in some ways the promise that treatment may be developed targeting genetically determined disease mechanism, pharmacogenomics.

The next 10–20 years will include both larger trials with more publicly available data and predefined subgroup analyses of these trials to try to determine which patients, based on their genetic makeups, are more likely to respond to particular therapies. The ultimate goal is the availability of more accurate data on the efficacy and safety of treatment and more comprehensive data on individual factors likely to affect a person's response to a treatment. Exciting science has made available agents that actually have major effects on rheumatic diseases and have placed us at this point where the future offers control of diseases that used to be both fatal and disabling.

## REFERENCES

1. Deyo RA, Diehl AK, Rosenthal M. How many days of bed rest for acute low back pain? A randomized clinical trial. N Engl J Med 1986;315:1064–1070.

2. Clements PJ, Furst DE, Wong WK, et al. High-dose versus low-dose D-penicillamine in early diffuse systemic sclerosis: analysis of a two-year, double-blind, randomized, controlled clinical trial. Arthritis Rheum 1999;42:1194–1203.

3. Moseley JB, O'Malley K, Petersen NJ, et al. A controlled trial of arthroscopic surgery for osteoarthritis of the knee. N Engl J Med 2002;347:81–88.

4. Boers M, Verhoeven AC, Markusse HM, et al. Randomised comparison of combined step-down prednisolone, methotrexate and sulphasalazine with sulphasalazine alone in early rheumatoid arthritis. Lancet 1997;350:309–318.

5. Keen HI, Pile K, Hill CL. The prevalence of underpowered randomized clinical trials in rheumatology. J Rheumatol 2005;32:2083–2088.

6. Felson DT, Anderson JJ, Boers M, et al. The American College of Rheumatology preliminary core set of disease activity measures for rheumatoid arthritis clinical trials. The Committee on Outcome Measures in Rheumatoid Arthritis Clinical Trials. Arthritis Rheum 1993;36:729–740.

7. Felson DT, Anderson JJ, Boers M, et al. American College of Rheumatology. Preliminary definition of improvement in rheumatoid arthritis. Arthritis Rheum 1995;38:727–735.

8. Yuen SY, Pope JE. Learning from past mistakes: assessing trial quality, power and eligibility in non-renal systemic lupus erythematosus randomized controlled trials. Rheumatology 2008;47:1367–1372.

# Chapter 26

# Methotrexate: Personal Reflections

**Michael E. Weinblatt**

*Brigham and Women's Hospital, Rheumatology and Immunology, Boston, MA*

The treatment of rheumatoid arthritis (RA) in the 1980s used a pyramid approach in which patients were started on anti-inflammatory drugs, primarily aspirin and nonsteroidal anti-inflammatory drugs, and then slowly escalated to a group of drugs called slow-acting antirheumatic drugs. This class of drugs included gold salts, hydroxychloroquine, and D-penicillamine, as well as immunosuppressive agents such as azathioprine and cyclophosphamide. Other elements of this treatment regimen were short-term hospitalizations, physical therapy, and liberal uses of corticosteroids both orally and as injection therapy.

While I was a rheumatology fellow from 1978 to 1980 at the Robert Brigham Hospital in Boston, the pyramid approach was used in most RA patients. At that time, the only new therapy available for our RA patients was D-penicillamine! Needless to say, disease in many of our patients progressed to cause severe joint damage that required orthopedic surgery. New treatment approaches, including such extreme measures as total nodal irradiation, thoracic duct drainage, and plasmapheresis, were generally unsuccessful.

Providing the opportunity for more hope, however, were uncontrolled reports on the successful use of low-dose weekly methotrexate in RA. Gubner and colleagues in 1951 reported that aminopterin, which is the parent compound of methotrexate, worked in an open study in patients with rheumatoid arthritis and psoriasis [1]. For unexplained reasons, the rheumatology community did not seem interested in

*The ACR at 75: A Diamond Jubilee*
Copyright © 2009 by John Wiley & Sons, Inc.

studying methotrexate for the treatment of RA. Part of this situation might be attributable to the enthusiasm in the rheumatology community in the 1950s for corticosteroids. Furthermore, rheumatologists were significantly concerned about the toxicity of methotrexate. A few pioneering community rheumatologists including Rex Hoffmeister in Spokane and Robert Willkens in Seattle observed improvement in RA activity with low-dose weekly methotrexate.

When I completed my fellowship in 1980, I became interested in studying methotrexate as a treatment of RA, having been attracted by reports from Hoffmeister and Willkens and the experience with methotrexate in psoriasis and psoriatic arthritis. There was great interest from my colleagues at the Brigham including Jon Coblyn, Pat Fraser, and Ron Anderson to pursue this study as well as interest among my research colleagues (David Glass, David Trentham, and David Fox) in performing mechanistic studies. In 1982, I submitted a protocol to Lederle Laboratories, the manufacturer of methotrexate, to support this trial. Several weeks later, they informed me that they were not currently interested in supporting studies of methotrexate in rheumatoid arthritis but would keep the protocol on file.

Approximately 6 months later, the group at Lederle asked if I could attend a meeting in Pearl River, New York, to discuss the protocol. To this day, I still do not know why they changed their minds and decided to support studies in RA, particularly because methotrexate was by then a generic drug. Also attending that meeting were Jim Williams and John Ward from the University of Utah who were the directors of the Cooperative Systematic Studies of Rheumatic Disease (CSSRD) Program and Joel Kremer from Albany Medical College. The CSSRD had a protocol for randomized placebo controlled study, and Joel Kremer wanted to conduct a prospective open study of methotrexate on the effects of methotrexate on the liver.

We submitted our formal protocol to Lederle for a 35-patient, 24-week placebo controlled study with a budget in the range of $95,000! In addition to financial support, Lederle provided drug and blinded placebo tablets. We started our study in 1983 and published our results in 1985 [2]. Both our study and the CSSRD study demonstrated the effectiveness of low-dose weekly methotrexate in patients with active rheumatoid arthritis [2,3]. These two studies were the pivotal studies submitted by Lederle Laboratory to the Food and Drug Administration for approval of methotrexate in rheumatoid arthritis.

When randomized trial was completed, our patients entered a long-term extension study [4], which paralleled the long-term studies of Joel Kremer [5]. In fact, both of our long-term studies exceeded 11 years of clinical observation.

Jim Williams and I presented our trials to the Arthritis Advisory Committee of the Food and Drug Administration in 1986. Most of the morning session was a discussion of the possible risk of malignancies associated with immunosuppressive therapies including azathioprine and cyclophosphamide. Methotrexate was not associated with either a higher risk of primary solid malignancies or recurrent malignancy. The afternoon session included a review of the pivotal studies and discussions on hepatic and pulmonary toxicity. At the conclusion of the session, the Arthritis Advisory Committee overwhelmingly recommended in favor of the approval of methotrexate for patients with active rheumatoid arthritis.

Following the initial placebo-controlled studies, subsequent clinical trials compared methotrexate to other disease-modifying therapies. These studies included patients who had not received prior gold salt therapy, providing a population of patients who were relatively treatment naïve and had earlier disease. These comparison studies included oral gold, intramuscular gold and azathioprine. Following completion of these comparative studies, combination studies were conducted in the late 1980s and early 1990s combining methotrexate with antimalarials, sulfasalazine, gold salts, auranofin, azathioprine, cyclosporine, and early biologic-response modifiers, including anti-CD4 therapy.

Many investigators were interested in learning more about the toxicity profile of the drug and in developing strategies to reduce side effects. Sarah Morgan and Graciella Alarcon were instrumental in performing studies on the use of folic acid to reduce toxicity. Harriet Kiltie at Lederle Laboratory was extremely supportive of sponsoring studies on the effects of methotrexate on the liver and lung. Data generated from the studies of serious liver disease and methotrexate was used by an American College Rheumatology (ACR) subcommittee to develop the guidelines on monitoring for liver toxicity.

Over the years, there has also been significant interest in identifying the mechanisms of action of this drug in RA with major contributions from the laboratory of Bruce Cronstein.

Complementing the work done in the United States and Canada, Rolf Rau in Germany conducted studies that compared methotrexate with gold and also performed some initial radiographic studies to show slowing of radiographic progression with methotrexate. The development program of methotrexate, which was started first by community and then academic rheumatologists in North America, became a truly international effort. Great camaraderie existed among the researchers in North America and Europe to pursue important clinical questions on this drug.

With the approval of methotrexate in the late 1980s, interest and enthusiasm gradually increased for the use of methotrexate in RA. Twenty years later, methotrexate has now become the most widely used therapy for the treatment of rheumatoid arthritis. Part of the enthusiasm for methotrexate relates to the validation of its efficacy in the studies of the biologic response modifiers and the observation that most biologics [anti-tumor necrosis factor (anti-TNF), rituximab, and abatacept] work better in combination with methotrexate than as mono therapy.

It has been personally gratifying to participate in the initial development of this drug and to observe the tremendous interest that remains in methotrexate even 25 years after the first studies. Methotrexate has now become the standard of care for patients with rheumatoid arthritis and juvenile idiopathic arthritis. Methotrexate is a major advance in the therapy of rheumatoid arthritis.

## REFERENCES

1. Gubner R, August S, Ginsberg V. Therapeutic suppression of tissue reactivity. II. Effect of aminopterin in rheumatoid arthritis and psoriasis. Am J Med Sci 1951;22:176–182.

2.  Weinblatt ME, Coblyn JS, Fox DA, et al. Efficacy of low-dose methotrexate in rheumatoid arthritis. N Engl J Med 1985;312:818–822.
3.  Williams HJ, Willkens RF, Samuelson CO, Jr., et al. Comparison of low-dose oral pulse methotrexate and placebo in the treatment of rheumatoid arthritis. A controlled clinical trial. Arthritis Rheum 1985;28:721–730.
4.  Weinblatt ME, Trentham DE, Fraser PA, et al. Long-term prospective trial of low-dose methotrexate in rheumatoid arthritis. Arthritis Rheum 1988;31:167–175.
5.  Kremer JM, Lee JK. The safety and efficacy of the use of methotrexate in long-term therapy for rheumatoid arthritis. Arthritis Rheum 1986;29:822–831.

Chapter *27*

# *Reflections on the Evolution of Anti-TNF Therapy: A Journey of Discovery*

### Ravinder Nath Maini

*Kennedy Institute of Rheumatology, Imperial College School of Medicine,*
*Hammersmith, London, England*

### Marc Feldmann

*Kennedy Institute of Rheumatology, Cytokine Biology and Immunology, London, UK*

## 27.1 IMMUNOLOGICAL ANTECEDENTS

### 27.1.1 R.N. Maini: Soluble Mediators of Delayed Hypersensitivity

I was propelled into the laboratory as a research Fellow in 1968 by curiosity about mechanisms of disease and especially the fascinating role of autoimmunity in rheumatoid arthritis (RA). By that time, the pathology of RA had been well described, with the presence of rheumatoid factor and immunoglobulin and depletion of complement in joints lending credibility to the concept of an immune complex mediated autoimmune pathogenesis [1]. Convinced that the emerging role of lymphocytes was an exciting new avenue to explore, I embarked on my studies with Dudley Dumonde, my immunological supervisor, at The Kennedy Institute, London.

My experiments in humans resulted in the demonstration of a biological activity called "lymphocyte mitogenic factor" in supernatants of lymphocytes cultured with

*The ACR at 75: A Diamond Jubilee*
Copyright © 2009 by John Wiley & Sons, Inc.

tuberculin, from normal subjects with a positive, but not those with a negative, skin-delayed hypersensitivity test to tuberculin. The factor joined Migration Inhibition Factor [2], in a class of intercellular messenger molecules produced by lymphocytes named "lymphokines" by the Dumonde group. Although my results were published in *Nature*, the problems of standardization of assays, failed attempts at the biochemical characterization of the factors, and an emerging plethora of other pre-formed, or synthesized, biologically activities produced by lymphocytes (dependent or independent of antigen), attested to the complexity of the field [3]. Soon afterward, it became clear that such factors were also produced by monocytes and other cell types, and the term "cytokines" was added to the dictionary.

Realizing that it would be impossible to apply the rudimentary knowledge of the biology of cytokines to studies of clinical relevance in RA, my focus of research took a new direction. Jerry Lawrence at New York University had described an entity termed transfer factor (TF) in the low-molecular-weight and dialyzable fraction of extracts of lymphocytes, which transferred specific delayed hypersensitivity. Dumonde and I speculated that depressed skin delayed hypersensitivity tests to several bacterial and fungal antigens in RA reflected a cell-mediated immune deficiency correctable by leukocyte dialyzates, putatively rich in TF, from healthy donors, and a small placebo-controlled "cross-over" study was performed in RA. The results were disappointing, with no demonstrable clinical efficacy distinguishable after TF and placebo administration. The *in vitro* laboratory tests were too variable over time to be interpretable. Both groups of patients showed an enhancement of skin hypersensitivity reactions when repeating the skin tests; however, this was likely a consequence of repeated skin tests [4]. Attempts to characterize TF as a molecular entity were unsuccessful, and my interest in it waned.

With the subsequent emergence of regulatory and ethical issues involved in the management of clinical trials, it is clear that it would be impossible for such a clinical trial to be undertaken in an academic setting today. In retrospect, my involvement in such studies seemed naïve, but immunological clinical science was largely phenomenological and inexact at this stage. As described later, I returned to work in the field of cytokines when it came of age a decade later and then prospered. However, the lack of progress in the early years was not entirely nonproductive because the strengths and weaknesses of clinical and laboratory measurements proved to be of value in the incremental advances that I applied to clinical research in my career.

### 27.1.2  M. Feldmann: Preparation for Molecular Discovery

My Ph.D. training generated many interests and skills that were very helpful for the codiscovery and development of anti-tumor necrosis factor (anti-TNF) therapy. The training took place at the Walter and Eliza Hall Institute (WEHI) 10 years after Sir Frank McFarlane Burnet [5] had clearly enunciated the concept of autoimmunity and autoimmune diseases. Thus, from my entry into research, understanding the mechanism of autoimmunity and autoimmune diseases was a "holy grail."

My Ph.D. project was to optimize immune cell survival and growth *in vitro* to facilitate to the measurement of a spectrum of immune phenomena *in vitro*, so that the cellular and molecular details could be investigated in depth. One aspect of my Ph.D. work was investigating mechanisms of cell interactions. In 1968, Jacques

Miller and his colleagues published a landmark series of papers [6] documenting that thymus-derived (subsequently T cell) and bursa or bone-marrow derived (subsequently B cells) interacted to produce antibody. How these rare cells, which were antigen specific, interacted or "collaborated" was not known. Cell contact vied with the role of intercellular mediators as potential mechanisms. With a medical background, where hormones were well characterized powerful signals that regulate many key life events such as growth and reproduction, I favored the intercellular mediators.

### 27.1.3  M. Feldmann: Rationale for Seeking a Molecular Trigger

In the 1980s after a decade of exploring immune regulation *in vitro* with mouse cells and subsequently human cells, I decided to study human immunological disease. The commonest problem in human immunology is the weak or nonexistent immune response to cancer. I thought that understanding how the immune system could be used to fight cancer might emerge from understanding the diseases where the immune system attacks the body, which are called autoimmune diseases.

While exploring the molecular mechanisms of autoimmunity was contemplated in the early 1980s, it was accelerated by that well-known ally of science, serendipity, which is not quite accurately simplified as "good luck." University College, where I worked in London, was 5 minutes from the Middlesex Hospital Department of Immunology, where Franco Bottazzo worked; Franco was a protégé of Deborah Doniach and Ivan Roitt, who had identified autoantibodies to thyroid. With Ricardo Pujol-Borrell and Toshi Hanafusa, Franco had been performing immunofluorescence studies of thyroid disease tissue. He was keen to discuss the recent findings of expression of human leukocyte antigen (HLA) class II molecules (HLA-DR) in both types of autoimmune thyroiditis, Graves' disease, and Hashimoto's thyroiditis on epithelial cells. Having worked since my PhD on cell interactions, including between macrophages and T lymphocytes, it seemed that if HLA-DR, which is the recognition structure for $CD4^+$ T cells, was present, then these epithelial cells might be capable of antigen presentation and triggering autoimmune T cells.

The upregulation of the major histocompatibility complex (MHC) in RA had also been described, and augmented antigen presentation might to be a common thread. In 1983, I wrote a hypothesis to connect HLA expression and molecular mechanisms of autoimmunity with upregulated antigen presentation and cytokines as key [7]. Testing that hypothesis, starting in 1983, paved the way for our work on molecular pathogenesis of RA.

## 27.2  AGE OF ENLIGHTENMENT

### 27.2.1  R.N. Maini: The Journey from Bench to Bedside

In the 1980s, protein purification and DNA technology made spectacular inroads into the cloning and expression of recombinant cytokines, such as interferons, interleukins, and tumor necrosis factor and their receptors. The simultaneous availability of specific monoclonal antibodies and complementary DNA (cDNA) probes, for the first time, made it possible for my laboratory to undertake studies on the role of cytokines in health and disease on cells and tissues from patients and experimental animal models. Later on, methods for producing monoclonal antibodies and receptor fusion proteins at industrial level were developed. We were fortunate that chimeric antibody technology had been harnessed and enabled our therapeutic study in 1992. Today, humanized, fully human and antibody fragments are a major class of new drugs being developed for the treatment of immune-inflammatory diseases.

The impact of the "new" technology on the role of cytokines on concepts of pathogenesis of RA was significant. By the early 1980s, credible evidence had emerged that purified interleukin-1 (IL-1) and TNFα were potentially arthritogenic. Notably, Jean-Michel Dayer observed that these two cytokines could induce the production of prostaglandin-E2 and collagenase (both recognized mediators of inflammation) by macrophages and synovial cells *in vitro*; Jerry Saklatvala demonstrated their role in destruction of cartilage in an organ culture model and their proinflammatory properties by intra-articular injection into normal rabbit joints. Marc Feldmann's hypothesis on the key role of cytokines in autoimmune disease added to my conviction that our skills were complementary and discussions with him led to our first joint project.

There are many answers to the question, "What led to a successful collaboration that resulted in the discovery of anti-TNF therapy?" First, that Marc and I experienced the same zeitgeist that was the basis of mutual understanding and trust; second, a shared enthusiasm for new ideas and innovation in the study of human disease; and third, the good fortune of a working with a joined up team of many talented young clinicians and laboratory scientists as well as the generous support of external collaborators.

Because we have extensively written on the "bench to bedside" history of the identification of TNF as a therapeutic target and development of anti-TNF therapy [8–10], here I will highlight the progress of only some of our work and lessons learned that have not received much attention before.

We began with the belief that the best way to investigate the pathogenesis of disease was to concentrate on studies of joint tissues from RA, and we proceeded to collect synovial tissue from surgical synovectomies and joint replacements. My research fellows were trained in arthroscopy and provided synovial biopsies form different stages of the disease for experimental studies; in addition, Ken Muirden from Melbourne, Australia, during a sabbatical visit, taught us how to obtain and examine pannus-cartilage junction tissue from surgical or cadaveric specimens for microscopic studies.

Several important results were obtained by immunohistological studies into the cellular source and range of cytokines produced in RA. Of particular significance was the finding by that TNFα was predominantly expressed by cells bearing macrophage markers in contrast to the expression of TNF-receptors by many cell types in the synovial and cartilage-pannus tissues. These data explained the pleiotropic biological effects of TNFα on the vasculature, synoviocytes, and immune-inflammatory cells in the local microenvironment of the joint and anticipated later findings in mechanism of action studies [11].

Synovial tissues were also used in experiments initiated in the Feldmann laboratory, which demonstrated the regulation of cytokine production in RA in an *in vitro* model. Cultures of enzymatically disaggregated synovial tissue cells maintained over several days spontaneously (without stimulants) produced IL-1, TNFα, IL-6 and granulocyte monocyte colony stimulating factor (GM-CSF). The production of IL-1 was abrogated by the addition of a specific antibody that neutralized the bioactivity of TNFα, and in later work this was shown to be true also for IL-6 and GM-CSF. These data established the concept that the chronically activated cytokine network in RA is maintained by autonomous signals dominated by TNFα.

Proof of concept that TNFα was indeed a therapeutic target was supported by studies in animal models and ultimately in successful clinical trials in RA, especially when there is an inadequate response to methotrexate and anti-TNF biologicals are added. Long-term, continuing treatment is necessary, suggesting that TNF production is downstream of as yet unknown irreversible pathways of TNF production. The exception to this rule has now been observed with a "legacy effect" of anti-TNF when it is used concomitantly with methotrexate in early RA; in this setting, it proves possible for it to be withdrawn with continuing control of disease activity. Our anti-TNF clinical trials also established an important principle that is applicable to successful biological drugs in immunologically mediated chronic diseases in general, that efficacy is related to the persistence of effective concentrations in blood and determines the frequency and dose of the drug. Additionally, the demonstration in RA patients that blockade of cell recruitment from the circulation into an inflammatory site, and partial restoration of homeostasis of the cytokine network, are major modes of action of anti-TNF therapy, likely applies to ankylosing spondylitis, psoriatic arthritis, psoriasis, and Crohn's disease.

### 27.2.2  M. Feldmann: Aspects of Working Together

I have had the privilege of collaborating with a wide range of scientists over the years (Figure 27.1). It has been an educational, enlightening, and empowering experience. Educational, as the very best teacher is a collaborator who needs to get you up to speed to enhance the collaboration. Enlightening, as paraphrasing the words of Donald Rumsfeld, the greatest unknowns are the ones that one could not even imagine existing. Empowering, as is summarized in the proverb "two heads are better than one." Science is intensely personal, and scientists are fiercely competitive about who gets the credit. This latter is well known, even to nonscientists.

So how is this reconciled? Collaborations are the quickest way to augment the skill and knowledge in a project. But the cost is shared credit. So the maintenance of the collaboration depends on social factors as well as scientific. Collaborators often turn into friends. If collaboration works, the returns can be much higher, as the productivity is greater. This was the case with Ravinder Maini and anti-TNF.

Loyalty to the group effort is essential for long-term success in a collaborative effort. If there are two or more divided "camps," then it would be much harder to sustain. We were fortunate that this was the case in the anti-TNF work, which was enhanced by the relatively early clinical success.

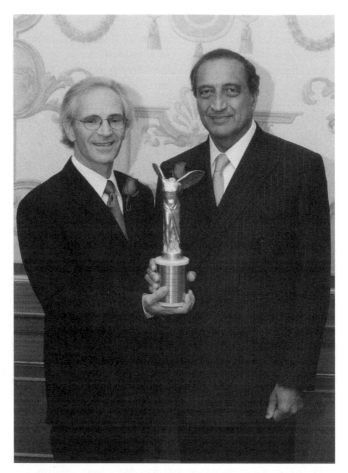

**FIGURE 27.1.** *Marc Feldmann and Ravinder Maini with the Albert Lasker Clinical Medical Research Award, 2003, "for discovery of anti-TNF therapy as an effective treatment for rheumatoid arthritis and other autoimmune diseases". (www.laskerfoundation.org/awards/2003clinical)*

### 27.2.3 Division of Labor

Academia is good at defining drug targets. Industry is good at developing drugs. True or false? Both are usually false, but a problem is the widespread belief that they are true.

Why should academia be good at defining drug targets? The "selection" process, in the Darwinian sense, for academics is for getting grants, as promotion without grants is hard to conceive. So, in academics, discovery research leads to proliferation of potential targets, the more the merrier, and not selection among potential targets.

Over 200 years ago, Adam Smith described a company as a "machine for making money [12]." So is it surprising that profitability, share holder value is what matters most? So a real problem in the pharmaceutical industry is the ratio of real innovation to minor increments. Many pharmaceutical developments are the latter. I was a witness to the rapid switching of anti-TNF biologics from sepsis to RA after the amazing results of our initial clinical trials were announced: a rational positive response to new data. But, as we visualize the anti-TNF market expanding, now (or soon will be) 5 contenders will each be fighting for market share.

Although this competition could seem to be good for the "consumer" or patients, is it really? Yes, more choices are available in terms of dosing. But what matters to patients and society most, the cost/benefit ratio has not changed. All the drugs are sold for roughly the same price. The pharmaceutical industry feels that cheaper drugs are always recognized to be less good, and so the industry leaders cannot recognize the point of trying to emulate Adam Smith's "bell shaped curve" to optimize the value of sales.

So the financial motives for companies to develop drugs can hinder real progress. The marketers know the value of existing markets but do not know the value of markets yet to be created. So they hinder risk taking into new areas of unknown value.

But what about the medical end of development: clinical trials? Are companies good at that? Yes and no. They are good at the highly complex technical process of performing the large-scale trials needed for the combined safety and efficacy analysis which is called a phase III registration trial. But are they good at small proof-of-principle trials, which help understand whether blocking a novel pathway has occurred, and has the hoped for beneficial result? This is a tall order, as companies do not have the required medical specialists/experts in all the appropriate fields: It would not make sense. The reality of optimizing drug development is to have significant and effective collaborations between those that have the novel molecules (companies) and the relevant expertise (academics). Better collaboration should reduce the cost of generating novel, safe and effective new medicines.

Did this happen with anti-TNF? To some extent it did. Anti-TNF therapy for RA started as an academic collaboration between R.N. Maini, M. Feldmann and Centocor scientists led by J.N. Woody. This is described in some detail in *Annual Reviews of Immunology* [13].

## 27.3  POSTSCRIPT

### 27.3.1  M. Feldmann: Can this Journey Guide Other Ventures?

Anti-TNF is the first major commercial success for "biologicals," which now include monoclonal antibodies and related molecules, as well as receptor Fc fusion proteins; sales were over $17 billion in 2008. This has had an impact on all big pharmaceutical companies, whose aversion to nonoral drugs was clear in the 1980s and 1990s, being convinced that the orally available organic chemicals with which they were familiar would always dominate the market over injectables. Now, almost half of clinical trials involve injectable "biologicals." The reasons seem clear: The toxicity of the biologicals, whose design mimics the body's own defence molecules (antibodies), is mechanism related; the large surface area of binding of antibodies and receptors with the target makes the unexpected binding and hence toxicity of small molecules rare.

A second aspect is the choice of therapeutic target. These need to be rate-limiting steps in the disease process but not in normal health or physiology. Many potential targets are risky. I feel strongly that cytokines (and their receptors) are good therapeutic targets, which exhibit many desired properties for therapeutic targets. Although our work with TNF blockade first demonstrated the power and utility of cytokine blockade, there have since been many other such examples. These include IL-1, IL6 blockade, and receptor activator of nuclear factor kappa B ligand (RANK-L) blockade. But it should not be assumed that such powerful drugs are necessarily safe. Although there are few nonspecific toxicities caused by binding to non-TNF or other cytokine targets, there are mechanism-related toxicities for all anticytokine therapeutics.

The benefit/risk ratio is relatively favorable, but because cytokines are pleiotropic (do many different things on diverse targets), their blockade is always liable to have affects apart from amelioration of the disease process. Because of the pleiotropic effects of cytokines and the genetic heterogeneity of the patient population, the range of potential toxicities is bewilderingly extensive. Nevertheless, what matters on a population basis is the frequency of these toxicities. The most frequent serious toxicity of anti, TNF is tuberculosis, which has a frequency of 1/2000 if no preventive screening is undertaken [14]. Is that high or low? In the light of the importance of TNF in host defense to intracellular organisms, it seems to many to be low. Certainly, this frequency is low enough not to deter usage. With appropriate screening, this figure is lowered 5–10-fold. Other severe infections also occur however less abundantly.

### 27.3.2 M. Feldmann and R.N. Maini: What is the Point of Mechanism of Action Studies?

Considerable evidence suggests that many therapeutics do not work in the way that was anticipated. The failure of a therapeutic to exert benefit despite mediating the expected effect can be helpful, misleading, or lead to a deeper understanding of the underlying biology. For example, in clinical trials of a anti-CD4+ monoclonal antibody, the marked depletion of circulating CD4+ cells was observed without associated clinical benefit. Whereas the conclusion that continued use of CD4+ T-cell depletion as a marker of response in early stage of drug development was not helpful, the argument against a role for T cells in RA was misleading as proven by the success of abatacept [CTLA4 immunoglobulin (Ig)], which blocks T cell activation. With increasing knowledge of the complex imbalance of CD4+ effector and regulatory subpopulations in RA, we can now propose why pan-CD4 depletion may have been ineffective.

If the therapeutic has the anticipated but incomplete clinical effect, then analyzing how it works may guide ways to improve efficacy and minimize risk. For example, the halting of bone erosions following anti-TNF therapy is more marked than its effect on signs and symptoms, and it argues for a differential mechanism. Because mechanism-of-action studies reveal that cell recruitment and angiogenesis are reduced but not abolished by TNF blockade, cotherapy targeting angiogenesis may augment efficacy.

Risk of infection could be minimized by seeking methods of blocking TNF-mediated pathways that target inflammatory but not host defense mechanisms.

Regrettably, unraveling the mechanism of action in detail is an elusive goal, but that should not act as a deterrent to learning as much as ethics and current technology will permit. It is an opportunity worth taking, as the study of therapeutic action provides one of the few approaches of studying pathophysiology of human disease.

## ACKNOWLEDGMENTS

The work described in this personal review was very ably assisted by many invaluable and talented colleagues over very many years.

*Pre–Clinical*
Fionula Brennan, Brian Foxwell, Ewa Paleolog, Andrew Cope, Peter Charles, Claudia Monaco, Richard Williams

*Clinical*
Peter Taylor, Michael Elliott (UK)
Jochen Kalden, Ferry Breedveld, Josef Smolen, Lars Klareskog (Europe)
Peter Lipsky (USA)

**Generous funding by:**
Arthritis Research Campaign, Kennedy Institute of Rheumatology Trustees, Wellcome Trust, Medical Research Council, Centocor Inc., Nuffield Foundation

## REFERENCES

1. Ziff M. Heberden Oration, 1964. Some immunological aspects of the connective tissues diseases. Ann Rheum Dis 1965;24:103–115.

2. Bloom BR, Jimenez L. Migration Inhibition Factor and the cellular basis of delayed-type hypersensitivity reactions. Am J Pathol 1970;60:453–466.

3. Dumonde DM, Maini RN. The clinical significance of mediators of cellular immunity Clin Allergy 1971;1:123–139.

4. Maini RN, Scott JT, Roffe LM, et al. Preliminary experience of transfer factor in rheumatoid arthritis: clinical and immunological studies. In: Infection, Immunology and the Rheumatic Disease. ( Dumonde DC, ed.). London UK: Blackwell Publications; 1975, p. 579–589.

5. Burnet FM. The Clonal Selection Theory of Acquired Immunity. Cambridge, UK: Cambridge University Press; 1959.

6. Miller JF, Mitchell GF. Cell to cell interaction in the immune response. I. Hemolysin-forming cells in neonatally thymectomized mice reconstituted with thymus or thoracic duct lymphocytes. J Exp Med 1968;128:801–820.

7. Bottazzo GF, Pujol- Borrell R, Hanafusa T, et al. Role of aberrant HLA-DR expression and antigen presentation in induction of endocrine autoimmunity. Lancet 1983;2:1115–1119.

8. Feldmann M, Brennan FM, Maini RN. Role of cytokines in rheumatoid arthritis. Annu Rev Immunol 1996;14:397–440.

9. Feldmann M, Maini RN. Anti-TNFα therapy of rheumatoid arthritis: What have we learned? Annu Rev Immunol 2001;19:163–196.

10. Feldmann M, Maini RN. TNF defined as a therapeutic target for rheumatoid arthritis and other autoimmune diseases. Nature Med 2003;9:1245–1250.

11. Maini RN, Feldmann M. How does infliximab work in rheumatoid arthritis? Arthritis Res 2002;4:S22–S28.

12. Smith A. An Inquiry into the nature and causes of the Wealth of Nations [ 3 vol.].: Dublin, Ireland: Whitestone; 1776.

13. Feldmann M. Translating molecular insights in autoimmunity into effective therapy. Annu Rev Immunol 2009;27:1–27.

14. Keane J, Gershon S, Wise RP, et al. Tuberculosis associated with infliximab, a tumor necrosis factor alpha-neutralizing agent. N Engl J Med 2001;345:1098–1104.

# Chapter 28

# NSAIDs: The Power of the Narrative

**Steven B. Abramson**

*Hospital for Joint Diseases/NYU, Department of Rheumatology/Medicine, New York, NY*

## 28.1 INTRODUCTION

This has been a remarkable time in the history of medicine, with the inception of molecular rather than empirical medicine, and our discipline of rheumatology has been at the forefront. At the end of the decade of the 1990s, the field was energized by the introduction of two classes of mechanism-based blockbuster drugs, tumor necrosis factor-alpha (TNFα) antagonists and Cyclooxygenase-2 (COX-2) selective agents. Although one class was to transform the treatment of rheumatoid arthritis, the other class was to transform not treatment but our views of the pharmaceutical industry, the Food and Drug Administration (FDA) and ourselves. The debate that ensued during this time regarding the use of nonselective versus selective Nonsteroidal Anti-inflammatory Drugs (NSAIDs), particularly related to the issue of cardiovascular risk, has been well covered in recent reviews and evidence-based treatment guidelines, such as those recently published by the Osteoarthritis Research Society International (OARSI) and the American College of Rheumatology (ACR) [1–3]. Therefore, this chapter will be more reflective and attempt to understand the remarkable modern history of NSAIDs, particularly the social and biomedical events that surrounded the introduction of the COX-2 inhibitors.

*The ACR at 75: A Diamond Jubilee*
Copyright © 2009 by John Wiley & Sons, Inc.

## 28.2   THE PERFECT STORM: UNDERSTANDING THE RISE AND FALL OF COX-2 INHIBITORS

Rheumatologists specialize in diseases often characterized by pain and inflammation, and they are well versed in the illustrious history surrounding the discovery and use of aspirin and related NSAIDs. Derived initially from willow bark, salicylate, and then aspirin have been used to treat inflammatory and noninflammatory pain for centuries. Aspirin became available in pill form in 1899, and as phenybutazone in 1949, and over 30 NSAIDs were subsequently introduced prior to the approval of the first COX-2 selective drugs, celecoxib and rofecoxib. During the decade of the 1990s, several transformative historical events converged to create a "perfect storm," which resulted in an unprecedented wave of enthusiasm for COX-2 inhibitors as a new class of "super aspirins." At least five independent occurrences provided the context for the rapid rise and the ultimate fall of the COX-2 inhibitors:

### 28.2.1   Computer Technologies and the Emergence of Medical Informatics

Beginning in the early 1990s, led by the groundbreaking analyses of the ARAMIS database by Fries et al. [4], NSAID-induced gastropathy emerged as an unexpectedly prevalent serious adverse event. Although gastrointestinal (GI) hemorrhage was a well-recognized risk of NSAID therapy, in the absence of large population data bases, the magnitude of the problem from a public health perspective — an estimated 100,000 hospitalizations and 15,000 deaths per year — was not. In the mid-1990s, as a result of compelling data reviewed publicly at a two-day meeting of the Arthritis Advisory Committee, the FDA added the "Black Box" GI warning to the NSAID class label. It was in this context that, quite independently, the new biology of COX-2 was beginning to emerge; the profession and the public could not have been better prepared for a new class of highly selective anti-inflammatory drugs, which were expected to be as effective as traditional NSAIDs but without their newly appreciated serious adverse GI events.

### 28.2.2   The Discovery of COX-2

Although NSAID-gastropathy provided the historical context for the success of COX-2 selective drugs in the marketplace, it was an interest in inflammation, not gastropathy, which led to the identification and characterization of the COX-2 isoform. Over several decades, prostaglandins had emerged as central mediators that cause inflammation and pain: First recognized in 1931 as a substance in semen that caused a female patient to have lower abdominal pain each time she had sexual intercourse, the substance was later named prostaglandin (*from the prostate gland*) by von Euler, and its biochemistry and biology was later characterized by Sune Bergström and Bengt Samuelsson. The fateful convergence of prostaglandins and NSAIDs resulted from the work of Sir John Vane, who identified prostacyclin and discovered that aspirin acted via the inhibition of the cyclooxygenase enzyme. In 1982, Noble prizes were awarded to Bergstrom, Samuelsson, and Vane for "for their discoveries concerning prostaglandins and related biologically active substances."

These discoveries were followed in 1992 by the identification of an endotoxin-inducible isoform of cyclooxygenase by Dr. Philip Needleman, who was then Senior Vice President of Monsanto and formerly the Chairman of the Department of Pharmacology at Washington University [5]. Needleman and colleagues set forth the hypothesis that soon became confirmed, that there were two enzymes existed: One a constitutive housekeeping enzyme and, the other an inducible form associated with inflammation. This discovery launched a rapid expansion of knowledge, which included not only the potential benefits of COX-1 sparing agents on platelets and the gastric mucosa but also an unanticipated potential role for COX-2 in reproduction, cancer, and Alzheimer's Disease [6].

From the perspective of many physicians and scientists, the identification of COX-2 in 1992 and the introduction of the COX-2 inhibitors to the clinic within 7 years represented a remarkable validation of "mechanism-based medicine" that had characterized the expectations of the prior decade. The discovery of COX-2 and its new biology were indeed considered breakthroughs — and the protagonists on the world stage, which included leading scientists in the field of eicosanoid biology, inflammation, and NSAID action — John Vane, Bengt Samuelsson, Phil Needleman, and Gerald Weissmann — were brilliant investigators of keen and engaging intellect. Among them were two Nobel laureates and one Knight of the British Empire (Figure 28.1). The fact that the exhilaration shared by physicians and scientists over the exciting biology of the cyclooxygenases was not demarcated by boundaries between industry and academia was another remarkable feature of the time, one that would arguably lead to insufficient scrutiny by the academic community when the focus of industry advanced from discovery to marketing.

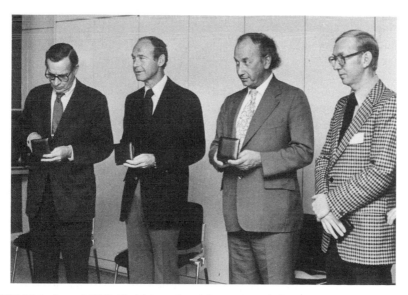

**FIGURE 28.1.** *August 1978. First International Congress on Inflammation held to celebrate the 900th anniversary of the founding of the University of Bologna. Shown are Lewis Thomas, Gerald Weissmann, John Vane and Bengt Samuelsson, receiving the Gold Medal of the University of Bologna.*

## 28.2.3   The Advent of Large Randomized Clinical Trials

Prior to 1990, most clinical trials in rheumatology included several hundred patients, and principal investigators were often university based. Landmark studies by leaders in rheumatology — Wilkens, Willliams, Kremer, and Weinblatt — led to the approval of methotrexate for the treatment of rheumatoid arthritis [7]. Since that time, however, because of increases in trial size and duration (coupled with the advances in computer technology that allow the analyses of large databases), phase III trials have become increasingly expensive and difficult to design and run. These changes resulted in the shift of clinical research from university-based investigators to industry. New drug applications (NDAs) for the phase III programs are of such magnitude that they can only be performed with the resources and infrastructure of the pharmaceutical industry. Randomized trials that focused on safety rather than an efficacy required even larger numbers: 8,000 for Celecoxib Long-term Arthritis Safety Study (CLASS) and Vioxx Gastrointestinal Outcomes Research (VIGOR), and more than 18,000 for Therapeutic Arthritis Research and Gastrointestinal Event Trial (TARGET). An unanticipated consequence of these large clinical trials was the emergence of safety signals for adverse events of low occurrence, most notably the cardiovascular signal in VIGOR, which were not prespecified primary or secondary endpoints, and therefore for which the studies had not been powered.

The CLASS and VIGOR trials were requested by the FDA in response to requests by the sponsors to have the GI (Black Box) Class Warning removed from the label of celecoxib and rofecoxib, respectively. Although some have argued that it *should* have been expected, the cardiovascular signal that merged from VIGOR was largely unanticipated and, given the low number of absolute events and the fact that the study had not been powered to detect these events, justifiably debated. Additional reports, which include randomized clinical trials and population-based studies, corroborated by animal models, would appear over the 2 years after the publication of VIGOR, which would confirm the increased risk of cardiovascular (CV) adverse events for both COX-2 agents and nonselective agents [1,2,8].

A significant problem that emerged during this period relates to the role of physician authors in industry-sponsored studies, particularly with respect to the access to and analysis of data provided by the companies. Too often, physician authors did not fulfill expected requirements for authorship, which include involvement in trial design, analysis of original data and writing of the manuscripts (*Uniform Requirements for Manuscripts Submitted to Biomedical Journals: Writing and Editing for Biomedical Publication. Updated October 2008,* http://www.icmje. org/index.html). This threat to the integrity of authorship was particularly troublesome as it became apparent that several postapproval clinical studies, which were designed by marketing to advance sales, included authors who were not sufficiently involved in the trial. Known as "seeding" trials, the objectives of such trials are designed to market the drug; in one instance cited as an egregious but representative example, a manuscript was allegedly "ghost written" by industry, and the physician first author had no involvement in the study until the company presented him with the manuscript for publication [10].

### 28.2.4    Medical Education and Communication Companies (MECCs) and the Growth of Pharma-Sponsored Medical Education Programs

Drug companies now support most continuing medical education, medical conferences, and meetings of professional association [11]. Over the past decade, a new industry emerged to accommodate this activity, called MECCs, which help prepare and build the market through professional education. These for-profit companies, which are primarily financed by industry, put together educational programs presented in hospital grand rounds, national society meetings, and in freestanding CME presentations. In addition, they arrange industry-sponsored "speaker training" sessions for physicians on speaker bureaus and prepare various other teaching materials for physicians, such as education slide sets, Compact disks read only memory (CD ROMs) and web-based broadcasts. The MECCs thus provided an effective new vehicle to communicate the COX-2 story to physicians, and their relationship to pharmaceutical companies represented by a cadre of "*speaker-trained*" physicians (!) ensured that the story told would achieve clear marketing objectives.

### 28.2.5    Direct to Consumer (DTC) Advertising

The groundswell of physician support for the COX-2 inhibitors — exciting biology, diminished concern about GI adverse events — was more than matched by interest generated among patients by intensive DTC marketing. DTC advertising accelerated in 1997 when the FDA changed regulations and allowed the description of adverse events to be reduced to brief statements that are now familiar on most television pharmaceutical advertisements. Subsequently, the amount of money spent on DTC advertising increased from $220 million in 1997 to over $2.8 billion in 2002, much of which was directed to promoting the benefits of the COX-2 inhibitors. Indeed, it is of interest, heralding this trend, that Rufen, which is ibuprofen manufactured by Boots, was the first drug to be advertised on U.S. television in 1983.

## 28.3    CONCLUSION

Thus, the rapid rise of the COX-2 inhibitors is best understood in the context of the remarkable convergence of independent events during the decade of the 1990s. In such a setting, there was power in the narrative told by scientists, clinicians, and industry, each viewing the story from different vantage points but together each sharing the excitement brought by possibilities of molecular medicine. And therein lie the central lessons of the COX-2 story for physicians: the understanding that there is power in the narrative that we tell, that we should not be smitten by explanations of biological plausibility not fully supported by the data and, most importantly, that we must differentiate the narrative of medicine from that of drug marketing. As a profession, we must ensure that the narrative of medicine is not scripted by industry and that it is not corrupted by "speaker-training," conflicted medical CME companies, "ghost-written" publications, and seeded clinical studies.

## REFERENCES

1. Moskowitz RW, Abramson S, Berenbaum F, et al. Coxibs and NSAIDs—is the air any clearer? Perspectives from the OARSI/International COX-2 Study Group Workshop 2007. Osteoarthr Cartil 2007;15:849–856.
2. American College of Rheumatology. Recommendations for use of selective and non-selective nonsteroidal antiinflammatory drugs: an American College of Rheumatology white paper. Arthritis Rheum 2008;59:1058–1073.
3. Zhang W, Moskowitz RW, Nuki G, et al. OARSI recommendations for the management of hip and knee osteoarthritis, Part II: OARSI evidence-based, expert consensus guidelines. Osteoarthr Cartil, 2008;16:137–162.
4. Fries JF, Williams CA, Bloch DA, et al. Nonsteroidal anti-inflammatory drug-associated gastropathy: incidence and risk factor models. Am J Med 1991;91:213–222.
5. Masferrer JL, Seibert K, Zweifel B, et al. Endogenous glucocorticoids regulate an inducible cyclooxygenase enzyme. Proc Natl Acad Sci U S A, 1992;89:3917–3921.
6. Dubois RN, Abramson SB, Crofford L, et al. Cyclooxygenase in biology and disease. Faseb J, 1998;12:1063–1073.
7. Weinblatt ME, Kremer JM. Methotrexate in rheumatoid arthritis. J Am Acad Dermatol, 1988;19:126–128.
8. Funk CD, FitzGerald GA. COX-2 inhibitors and cardiovascular risk. J Cardiovasc Pharmacol 2007;50:470–479.
9. Lisse JR, et al. Gastrointestinal tolerability and effectiveness of rofecoxib versus naproxen in the treatment of osteoarthritis: a randomized, controlled trial. Ann Intern Med, 2003;139:539–546.
10. Hill KP, et al. The ADVANTAGE seeding trial: a review of internal documents. Ann Intern Med 2008;149:251–258.
11. Relman AS, Ross SS, Egilman DS, Separating continuing medical education from pharmaceutical marketing. JAMA, 2001;285:2009–2012.

# Chapter 29

# Imaging in Inflammatory Arthritis: A Personal View

**Paul Emery**

*Chapel Allerton Hospital, Academic Unit of Musculoskeletal Disease, Leeds, England*

## 29.1 IMAGING AT DIAGNOSIS

Sensitive imaging techniques that allow simultaneous visualization of both soft-tissue inflammation and osteitis have provided an opportunity to examine the initial lesions of inflammatory arthritis. With this approach, it became clear that synovitis with bony reaction, or MRI bone oedema (histologically, an osteitis), was present at the earliest times in patients destined to develop RA [1,2]. The joint swelling and synovitis showed two patterns. Thus, intrasynovial disease with reactive osteitis/erosions was characteristic of RA. In contrast, an enthesitis with osteitis at the insertion of these tendons/ligaments was typical of spondyloarthropathy, with synovitis proposed as secondary [3,4] These findings are shown in Figure 29.1.

### 29.1.1 Erosions at Baseline

Whereas testing for serological markers (e.g., auto-antibodies and acute phase reactants) has improved diagnosis, at an individual patient level, the laboratory is limited since up to 40% of patients who develop RA are negative for these markers. Furthermore, an even higher proportion of autoantibody negativity in patients occurs

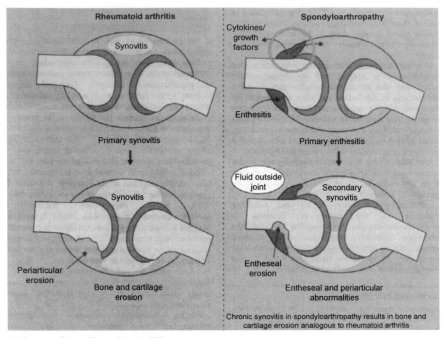

McGonagle, Gibbon, Emery, Lancet,1998.

**FIGURE 29.1.** *Diagrammatic representation of primary pathology of rheumatoid arthritis and spondyloarthropathy derived from sensitive imaging with MRI.*

in persistent undifferentiated arthritis; this condition is being increasingly recognized. However, the ability of imaging to provide evidence of synovitis as well as the bony reaction characteristic of RA makes these techniques virtually diagnostic for patients at presentation. Nevertheless, diagnosis needs to be interpreted in a clinical context, as synovitis with erosions can also be observed in polymyalgia rheumatica, which can usually be differentiated clinically [5].

This sensitivity of imaging is most relevant in early phases of disease because, after 12 weeks, the American College of Rheumatology (ACR) criteria are accurate for diagnosing RA [6]. For patients with a symptom duration of less than 12 weeks, however, RA can still be diagnosed with imaging. Moreover, an indication of prognosis can be achieved because early erosions predict more aggressive disease and long-term functional loss. Thus, imaging at baseline can provide an accurate diagnosis and prognosis, providing logic for more aggressive therapy.

## 29.1.2   Ultrasound (US)

Compared with MRI, which provides 3D tomographic imaging and bone visualization, US, which is more widely available, was originally regarded as too subjective for a reliable assessment tool in arthritis. The initial studies required the validation of ultrasound images that in turn led to improvements in reproducibility. In a study of early RA, Wakefield et al. [7] showed that erosions could be detected in around seven times as many patients using ultrasound as with X-ray. Furthermore, the data showed that plain X-rays were insensitive for measuring small erosions, which constituted 90% of those present in early disease [7] Figure 29.2.

Other studies have provided further validation for ultrasound in terms of measuring cortical breaks [8] and showed, that in patients treated with conventional therapy,

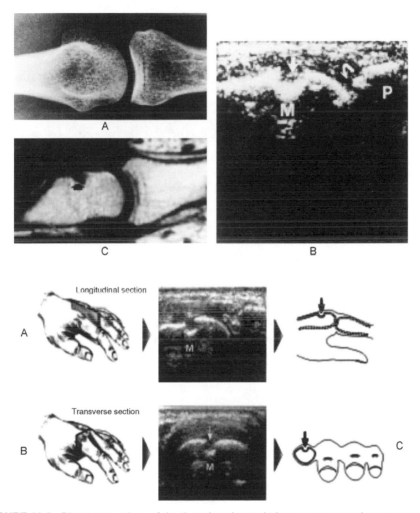

**FIGURE 29.2.** *Direct comparison of the three imaging techniques on a second metacarpophalangeal joint in a patient with early rheumatoid arthritis.* **A,** *Radiograph, showing normal results.* **B,** *Longitudinal sonographic image, demonstrating an erosion on the radial aspect of the second metacarpal head* **(M)** **(straight arrow). Curved arrow** *indicates joint space.* **C,** *Magnetic resonance imaging (T1-weighted spin-echo pulse sequence) coronal view, demonstrating bone marrow defect* **(arrow)** *corresponding to the same site as the sonographic erosion.* **P**= *phalanx.* **A,** *Longitudinal section through the second metacarpophalangeal joint, demonstrating a cortical defect* **(straight arrow)** *on the metacarpal head* **(M). Curved arrow** *indicates joint space.* **P**= *phalanx.* **B,** *Transverse section, confirming the defect as definite erosion.* **Straight arrows** *indicate identical sections in* **A** *and* **B** *on the schematic at right.*

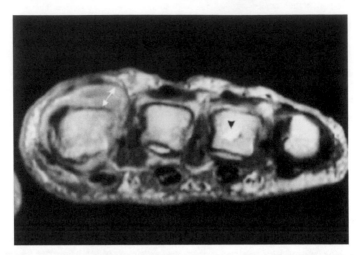

**FIGURE 29.3.** *Axial T1-weighted post-gadolinium sequences of the second through fifth metacarpophalangeal (MCP) joints. Before methotrexate and intraarticular corticosteroid (MTX + IAST) therapy. Marked MCP joint synovitis and tenosynovitis are visible, as demonstrated by high signal intensity.* **Arrow** *indicates the dimension measured for maximum synovial thickness.* **Arrowhead** *shows an erosion.*

the lesions seen on ultrasound and MRI were those that later became larger X-ray erosions [9] Figure 29.3. Another study demonstrated that biopsies of ultrasound erosions showed necrotic bone [10].

A major advantage of US over MRI is its ability to image multiple joints, which include hands and feet, at a single sitting. One study, assessing multiple joints in patients with early untreated oligoarthritis, demonstrated that one third of patients actually had a polyarticular disease [11]; of those who were rheumatoid factor (RF) positive, over 90% went on to fulfill ACR defined RA at 12 months. This finding suggests that techniques like US could provide important baseline assessment of early inflammatory patients.

### 29.1.3   Screening for Patients for Entry into Studies

In view of the limitations of plain radiographics, we felt that the application of MRI and US was valuable for disease monitoring and assessing disease mechanisms, including the possible uncoupling between inflammation and damage. For certain studies, particularly mode of action ones, imaging has become standard as an entry criterion, as patients are only included if they had synovitis with or without erosions. An example of such a study was that by Quinn et al. [12] which showed the increased statistical power of using a homogeneous study population in assessing a clinical response. Significant symptomatic benefits (ARC 20/50/70 improvement criteria) were documented for the more aggressive therapy of methotrexate and anti- tumour necrosis factor (TNF) over methotrexate monotherapy with only 20 patients; studies of heterogeneous rheumatoid arthritis patients would take several hundred to show such a difference. Another aspect of the study was the assessment of the benefits of early remission induction for the long-term outcome. It was shown that those patients who had remission induced and sustained for the first year (the latter was the case for all who achieved remission) could stop the biologic therapy and maintain their clinical state with just the standard DMARD (i.e., methotrexate). This study offered the first possibility of managing patients at a realistic cost. The principle was confirmed in the elegant BeST study [13].

## 29.2  ENTHESITIS

As noted, original MRI observations led to the hypothesis that the major pathology of the spondyloarthritides (SpAs) was entheseal in nature [4]. It also became clear that certain patients started with enthesitis, and over time, this lesion became intrasynovial and rheumatoid like. Now, studies have combined imaging with anatomy to increase understanding of the enthesis. This structure is now referred to as the enthesis organ, a concept that facilitates understanding the mechanobiology and the pathology of biomechanically induced inflammation [14,15].

## 29.3  IMAGING AT STABLE STATE

### 29.3.1  Synovitis and Damage

For many years, there was a debate about whether synovitis and damage are separate events whose distinct pathologies account for the disassociation observed in clinical trials. This issue has now been resolved by the use of imaging with ultrasound and MRI to measure synovitis and damage simultaneously. Although suggested before, in a landmark study, Conaghan et al. [16] showed that the level of synovitis in a joint correlated with subsequent damage in that individual joint (see Figure 29.4). Importantly, no joint without synovitis progressed. There was also a correlation between the amount of synovitis and the likelihood of damage, with 50% likelihood of damage in a joint a over a 9-month period if there was 5 mm or more of synovitis. This study made it clear that the aim of therapy should be to reduce synovitis. If this could be achieved, then the patient would safe from structural damage.

However, some patients with evidence of disease activity from the disease activity score (DAS) can have pain sensitization or fibromyalgia. In such patients, imaging can provide evidence that there is no synovitis and hence no risk of structural damage; in these patients, the aggressive use of biological therapies is probably not appropriate.

### 29.3.2  Remission on DMARDs

Supporting a dissociation between synovitis and clinical damage are the data showing that the patients in clinical remission can progress structurally [17]. Until better imaging was available, it was impossible to determine why this occurred. However, a

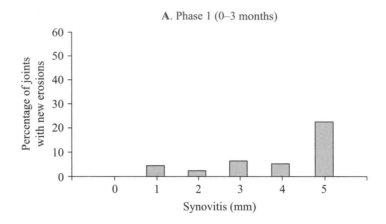

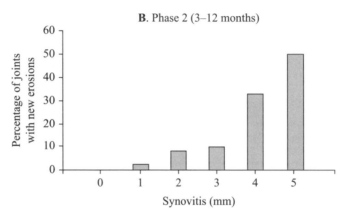

**FIGURE 29.4.** *Percentage of all joints with new erosions versus mean level of synovitis, during phase 1 (**A**) and phase 2 (**B**). Level of synovitis is rounded to the nearest whole number. Data are based on individual joint measurements.*

study by Brown et al. [18] on over 100 patients in clinical remission on DMARDs showed that virtually all patients had subclinical synovial thickening on MRI and ultrasound and that around half had evidence of more active synovitis with positive gadolinium enhancement and Power Doppler. The hypothesis moved from a disassociation between synovitis and structural damage to the existence of subclinical disease in patients in clinical remission. In a follow-up study, Brown et al. [19], provided data showing that the individual joints that had synovitis (with or without symptoms) had a greatly increased risk of progression (Figure 29.5).

A remaining question about remission concerns the basis for the structural benefits of TNF blockade. Preliminary data suggest that imaging findings of patients on TNF inhibitors or other DMARDs in remission do not differ significantly, which suggests that the structural benefits of TNF blockade may not relate entirely to the level of suppression of synovitis and that another mechanism (e.g., suppression of RANKL) may contribute [20]. However, it must be remembered TNF blockers induce remission

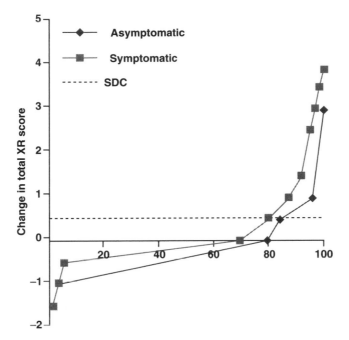

**FIGURE 29.5.** *Cumulative probability distribution of the percentages of symptomatic and asymptomatic patients with a given change in total radiographic (x-ray[XR]) score (smallest detectable change [SDC]).*

in a higher proportion of patients than conventional DMARDs. Of note in this respect, is a mode of action study showing that a powerful bisphosphate, which is zolendronic acid, can reduce erosions in patients on methotrexate by 90% [21].

**The Indicating Evolution of Evidence for Sensitive Imaging.**

1. US and MRI evidence of erosions in RA at disease onset with normal x-rays
2. Confirmation that MRI and US changes correspond to erosions
3. Demonstration that US and MRI changes predict later X-ray erosion
4. Demonstration that the level of synovitis predicts erosions in individual joints
5. Demonstration of imaging remission and the effects of DMARDs on this state
6. Explanation for progression of erosions in DMARD-induced remission
7. Elucidation of the relationship between pathologies for synovitis and erosion
8. Elucidation of pathologies of arthritis using imaging in early disease

## 29.4  WHEN TO IMAGE

Imaging patients with arthritis can be most instructive about pathology, diagnosis, and prognosis. Ultrasound is labor intensive, however, and MRI requires relatively costly equipment with sometimes limited availability. Therefore, to use imaging efficiently, it should be targeted to the times when critical information is needed. The times include the following: first, at presentation when there is doubt about diagnosis especially with short duration of symptoms; second, in patients entering in a mode of action study or being enrolled for aggressive therapy where accurate diagnosis and prognosis are crucial; and, third, when patients reach a stable state to predict the likelihood of additional structural damage.

The major advances of imaging in elucidating the pathogenesis of inflammatory synovitis are now being followed by insights into the pathology of spondyloarthropathies, including psoriatic arthritis [22] and osteoarthritis [23,24]. Furthermore, imaging other aspects of disease such as tendon disease [25] and the time course of response in inflammatory arthritis [26] is becoming increasingly important. The role of rheumatologists in providing an ultrasound service is also being clarified with a systematic review of the requirements for competency for the performance of these studies [27]. Finally, the technological advances such as dedicated extremity MRI will allow many studies to be performed at lower cost and greater convenience.

## ACKNOWLEDGMENTS

*Leeds Musculoskeletal Imaging Group*
Dennis McGonagle, Philip Conaghan, Richard Wakefield, Richard Reece, Doug Veale, Ai Lyn Tan, Maya Buch, Jane Freeston, Zunaid Karim, Andrew Brown, Mark Quinn, Mike Green, Philip O'Connor, Andrew Grainger, and Wayne Gibbon
*EULAR/OMERACT MRI Group*
Mikkel Ostergaard, Charles Peterfy, Fiona McQueen, Harry Genant, and Paul Bird
*EULAR/OMERACT Ultrasound Task Force*

## REFERENCES

1. McGonagle D, Conaghan PG, O'Connor P, et al. The relationship between synovitis and bone changes in early untreated rheumatoid arthritis: a controlled magnetic resonance imaging study. Arthritis Rheum 1999;42:1706–1711.

2. Ostergaard M, Hansen M, Stoltenberg M, et al. New radiographic bone erosions in the wrists of patients with rheumatoid arthritis are detectable with magnetic resonance imaging a median of two years earlier. Arthritis Rheum 2003;48:2128–2131.

3. McGonagle D, Gibbon W, O'Connor P, et al. Characteristic magnetic resonance imaging enthesea changes of knee synovitis in spondylarthropathy. Arthritis Rheum 1998; 41:694–700.

4. McGonagle D, Gibbon W, Emery P. Classification of inflammatory arthritis by enthesitis. Lancet 1998;352:1137–1140.

5. Marzo-Ortega H, Rhodes LA, Tan AL, et al. Evidence for a different anatomic basis for joint disease localization in polymyalgia rheumatica in comparison with rheumatoid arthritis. Arthritis Rheum 2007;56:3496–3501.

6. Green M, Marzo-Ortega H, McGonagle D, et al. Persistence of mild, early inflammatory arthritis: the importance of disease duration, rheumatoid factor, and the shared epitope. Arthritis Rheum 1999;42:2184–2188.

7. Wakefield RJ, Gibbon WW, Conaghan PG, et al. The value of sonography in the detection of bone erosions in patients with rheumatoid arthritis: a comparison with conventional radiography. Arthritis Rheum 2000;43:2762–2770.

8. Døhn UM, Ejbjerg BJ, Court-Payen M, et al. Are bone erosions detected by magnetic resonance imaging and ultrasonography true erosions? A comparison with computed tomography in rheumatoid arthritis metacarpophalangeal joints. Arthritis Res Ther 2006;8:R110.

9. McQueen FM, Benton N, Crabbe J, et al. What is the fate of erosions in early rheumatoid arthritis? Tracking individual lesions using x-rays and magnetic resonance imaging over the first two years of disease. Ann Rheum Dis 2001;60:859–868.

10. McGonagle D, Gibbon W, O'Connor P, et al. A preliminary study of ultrasound aspiration of bone erosion in early rheumatoid arthritis. Rheumatology 1999;38:329–331.

11. Wakefield RJ, Green MJ, Marzo-Ortega H, et al. Should oligoarthritis be reclassified? Ultrasound reveals a high prevalence of subclinical disease. Ann Rheum Dis 2004; 63:382–385.

12. Quinn MA, Conaghan PG, O'Connor PJ, et al. Very early treatment with infliximab in addition to methotrexate in early, poor-prognosis rheumatoid arthritis reduces magnetic resonance imaging evidence of synovitis and damage, with sustained benefit after infliximab withdrawal. Arthritis Rheum 2005;52:27–35.

13. Goekoop-Ruiterman, et al. Comparison of treatment strategies in early rheumatoid arthritis: a randomized trial. The Annals of Internal Medicine 2007;146:406–415.

14. Benjamin M, Moriggl B, Brenner E, et al. The enthesis organ concept — why enthesopathies may not present as focal insertional disorders. Arthritis Rheum 2004;50:3306–3313.

15. Benjamin M, Toumi H, Suzuki D, et al. Microdamage and altered vascularity at the enthesis — bone interface provides an anatomic explanation for bone involvement in the HLA-B27-associated spondylarthritides and allied disorders. Arthritis Rheum 2007; 56:224–233.

16. Conaghan P, O'Connor P, McGonagle D, et al. Elucidation of the relationship between synovitis and bone damage: a randomized MRI study of individual joints in patients with early RA. Arthritis Rheum 2003;48:64–71.

17. ten Wolde S, Breedveld FC, Hermans J, et al. Randomised placebo-controlled study of stopping second-line drugs in rheumatoid arthritis. Lancet 1996;347:347–352.

18. Brown AK, Conaghan PG, Karim Z, et al. An explanation for the apparent dissociation between clinical remission and continued structural deterioration in rheumatoid arthritis. Arthritis Rheum 2008;58:2958–2967.

19. Brown AK, Quinn MA, Karim Z, et al. Presence of significant synovitis in rheumatoid arthritis patients with disease-modifying antirheumatic drug-induced clinical remission: evidence from an imaging study may explain structural progression. Arthritis Rheum 2006;54:3761–3773.

20. Saleem B, Emery P. The remission state of patients treated with combination TNF blocker and DMARD therapy: A clinical and imaging comparative study. Arthritis Rheum, In press.

21. Jarrett SJ, Conaghan PG, Sloan VS, et al. Preliminary evidence for a structural benefit of the new bisphosphonate zoledronic acid in early rheumatoid arthritis. Arthritis Rheum 2006;54:1410–1414.

22. McGonagle D, Conaghan PG, Emery P. Psoriatic arthritis: A unified concept twenty years on. Arthritis Rheum 1999;42:1080–1086.

23. Tan AL, Grainger AJ, Tanner SF, et al. A high-resolution magnetic resonance imaging study of distal interphalangeal joint arthropathy in psoriatic arthritis and osteoarthritis: Are they the same? Arthritis Rheum 2006;54:1328–1333.

24. Tan AL, Grainger AJ, Tanner SF, et al. High-resolution magnetic resonance imaging for the assessment of hand osteoarthritis. Arthritis Rheum 2005;52:2355–2365.

25. Wakefield RJ, O'Connor PJ, Conaghan PG, et al. Finger tendon disease in untreated early rheumatoid arthritis: A comparison of ultrasound and magnetic resonance imaging. Arthritis Rheum 2007;57:1158–1164.

26. Wakefield RJ, Freeston JE, Hensor EMA, et al. Delay in imaging versus clinical response: A rationale for prolonged treatment with anti-tumor necrosis factor medication in early rheumatoid arthritis. Arthritis Rheum 2007;57:1564–1567.

27. Brown AK, O'Connor PJ, Wakefield RJ, et al. Practice, training and assessment amongst experts performing musculoskeletal Ultrasonography — towards the development of an international consensus of educational standards for Ultrasonography for rheumatologists. Arthritis Care Res 2004;51:1018–1022.

# Chapter *30*

# *Ethical Challenges of Modern Rheumatology*

**Richard S. Panush**

*Saint Barnabas Medical Center, Department of Medicine, Livingston, NJ*

---

### Author's Note

*I imagine a conversation about ethics with my mother who embodies the wisdom of the elders. She would say that ethics involves acting with honor, integrity, and respect, which underlie the principles of autonomy, distributive justice, and non-maleficence; that there is no entitlement by individuals or organizations for "gifts"; that "disclosure" is not acceptable; that subsidization for our education is unethical and unprofessional; that dishonorable individuals (like Reiter) should not be memorialized with eponymic recognition; and that affordable, safe, and efficient health care should be available to all. She would also say medicine needs an outcomes-based system where physicians practice without ethically conflicted incentives or disincentives. Finally, she would remind us to cherish our fundamental ethical and humanistic soul as we advance our art and science.*

---

"How are you, Ma? Ma, wake up!"

"Ah, it's you, son. I was awake, just reflecting. There's lots to remember at age 97. How's everybody? [1–3]"

"Rena still sings opera, and the kids are thriving—David's no longer certain that revolution is necessary, Jonathan still has his motorcycle, and Rachel has two adorable children: Lia, who wants to be a princess, and Etan, a truck driver [1–3]."

---

"And the dogs? You were fond of them."

"Well, Goldie, a certified nutritional consultant, and Tevye, her consort, known to many in rheumatology, died from lupus and Sjogren's syndrome, respectively. Now we have Sweedee, a certified (pet) therapist, whom David and I found abandoned when we were running, and Speckles, "rescued"from Puerto Rico, now living the American dream [4]."

"So, what have you been doing?"

"I'm trying to write about "ethical challenges of modern rheumatology" and can't get started. The editor wants something "lively," "personal," and "engaging." And not more than 1,000–1,500 words! Any ideas?"

"We can keep this short because lunch is pretty soon. Ethics is simple, son. Don't you remember anything from Sunday school? The Talmudic sages said there are three "crowns," or symbols of earthly accomplishment: learning, royalty, and priesthood; but the "crown" of a good name is the most exalted of all. They also said a man should make those choices that lead to honor. Ethics is really about behaving honorably and respecting individual dignity."

"What about the principles of ethics? Autonomy. Distributive justice. Non-maleficence. Beneficence [5,6]?"

"You don't think, son, what I just told you— respecting people and patients, acting honorably and treating others with dignity— encompasses this?"

"So, Ma, what does this mean for us in rheumatology?"

"Haven't we talked about gifts and industry relationships before? Didn't you once take a drug company-sponsored trip to Tahiti [8–10]?"

"That drug they were introducing seemed complicated then, like we needed a week in a secluded place to learn about it. And that happened a long time ago."

"Your father and I were not proud of that."

"I was different then and am still profoundly embarrassed about my behavior."

"You should be. You should not accept gifts. There's no entitlement to this. Where was it promised that someone else was supposed to provide for you, or offer you presents? And all these "gift" costs are passed on to patients, like me, without consent."

"Wouldn't disclosing gifts be acceptable?"

"No, son. Neither "disclosure" nor limiting gifts changes the ethical impropriety."

"Why, Ma?"

"Because medicine is a moral enterprise, linked to the highest ethical behavior. Accepting industry gifts is unethical, unprofessional, and unnecessary. Medicine is about dedication and devotion to patients even at personal and professional risk to profit, pride, and position [11–21]."

"What's so bad about a pen, or pizza, for the fellows or staff?"

"In addition to violating ethical precepts— unfairly allocating resources without patients' knowledge or consent— gifts obligate, son. Gifts influence behavior. Gifts erode physicians' role as trustees of patients' welfare, increasing costs of care, obligating physicians to companies. Also you learn much about prescribing from sources standing to profit from your choices [8–21]. Increasing numbers of thoughtful leaders, including the Association of American Medical Colleges, now advocate absolute prohibition of industry gifts [12,14,15,17–21]."

"Surely, Ma, we can resist inappropriate influences."

"Nonsense. You've told me about the robust data repeatedly documenting that this notion is wrong."

"So, Ma, if physicians shouldn't accept gifts, what about organizations? How can a society like the American College of Rheumatology (ACR) remain solvent if it stopped accepting corporate contributions?"

"Why should your professional organization have a different set of ethical expectations than its members? There is no organizational entitlement either. Why should members not pay for services they expect? Why should meetings be subsidized by industry? If members do not/will not support these expenses, then perhaps the organization should reconsider its activities and priorities."

"But, Ma, corporate contributions permit important organizational benefits— supporting fellows, research, advocacy, education, and scientific meetings. Member dues alone could not sustain these activities critical to the ACR, arguably to society and patients. And may not industry have a genuine, at least in part altruistic, stake in the future of rheumatology?"

"Do you really think, son, someone else should pay for your education— undergraduate, graduate, or continuing? Shouldn't that be your responsibility? The entire continuing medical education enterprise has become distorted. It desperately needs fixing."

"What do you think about eponyms, Ma? Wouldn't it be neat to have 'Panush's syndrome'?"

"Surely that's not the kind of recognition you seek, son. Perhaps it's time to move beyond eponyms [22,23]. Many are misattributed, some are silly, some obscure the relevant science, some led to payment denials, and some reflect reprehensible people like Reiter, a Nazi, complicit with atrocities; he certainly does not deserve eponymic recognition [24–26]."

"How about issues relating to health care, Ma, like managed care?"

"Managed care came about because of an ethical conflict inherent in the fee-for-service health care system. Before, the incentives were to provide the most care for the most number of patients for the most amount of money. With managed care, there's a similar ethical conflict in which the incentives are to do the least care on the least number of patients to make the most money. Neither system is satisfactory. The goal should be to accept managed care only as an inherently unstable transition because of the ethical conflicts involved. Medicine needs a system of outcomes-based, or evidence-based, health care in which physicians do the right amount of care on the right patients for the right reason [27,28]."

"Who pays for health care, Ma?"

"I know that equitable, accessible, affordable, and effective care should be a right available to all citizens. And how can physicians refuse to see patients for any reason? Medicine is a calling, not a business. Challenges will be to eliminate "waste," curtail costly care that is ineffective, assure physicians fulfill obligations to patients, and figure out how to ration limited resources equitably and ethically [27,28]."

"Ma, you're beginning to look fatigued, and we haven't even talked about clinical trials, investigators' relationships, consents, comparators, and availability of new and trial treatments yet."

"I am tired, son. I'm going to take a nap before I get my hair done. Next time let's talk about the family."

## ACKNOWLEDGMENTS

Sections of this imagined conversation were reprised from cited sources. Some drafts of and notes for the manuscript were written with generic pens and pencils on generic paper, perhaps to the disappointment of some. I spoke on some of these topics but received no honoraria or even travel reimbursements (the talks were local, however). My medical center still accepts occasional "unrestricted grants" for certain educational activities (my department doesn't), but we're working on that. My wife would have liked extra income from speakers' bureaus and consulting to reduce our mortgage, and my mom was embarrassed I drove an 11-year-old car, but I finally bought a hybrid. I miss my father, who died 2 years ago, and his wisdom. I miss the woman my mother once was too; she is no longer the articulate, thoughtful woman of my memory and imagination. Ironically, her decline was caused by a rheumatic illness. I have no doubt that, if she were knowledgeable about the ethical challenges confronting us and able to articulate her thoughts, she would have spoken as I conceived our conversation. And so would dad.

## REFERENCES

1. Panush RS. My son, the doctor. Amer J Med 1990;80:167–168.

2. Panush RS. My mother, the patient. Arthritis Rheum 1993;36:1754–1756.

3. Panush RS. My son, the chairman. J Clin Rheum 1995;1:245–248.

4. Panush RS, Levine M, Reichlin M. Do I need an ANA? Some thoughts about man's best friend and the transmissibility of lupus. J Rheum 2000;27:287–291.

5. Panush RS, Kavanaugh A, Romain P. Ethical issues in rheumatologic practice and investigation, Chapter 39, In Biological Therapy in Rheumatology., Smolen JS, Lipsky PE (eds). Martin Dunitz Publishers, London, UK 2003,pp. 639–651.

6. Dendi P, Desai S, Jacobs FM, et al. Why ethics are important to the busy practitioner caring for patients with rheumatologic and musculoskeletal disorders. Bull Rheum Dis 2003; 52:1–7.

7. Panush RS. Professionalism—it's all about the patient. And respect. Rounds. Saint Barnabas Health Care System. Winter 2003;1–2.

8. Panush RS. Not for sale, not even for rent: just say no. Thoughts about The American College of Rheumatology adopting a code of ethics. Viewpoint. J Rheumatol 2002; 29:1049–1057.

9. Panush RS. Reply (to Ellman MH: re "Not for sale, not even for rent: just say no. Thoughts about the American College of Rheumatology adopting a code of ethics"). J Rheumatol 2003;30:202–203.

10. Panush RS. Why I no longer accept pens (or other gifts) from industry (and why you shouldn't either). J Rheumato 2004;31:1478–1482.

11. Pellegrino ED, Relman AS. Professional medical associations. Ethical and practical guidelines. JAMA 1999;282:984–986.

12. Relman AS. Separating continuing medical education from pharmaceutical marketing. JAMA 2001;285:2009–2012.

13. Hadler NM. Hubris for sale or rent. Available at http://www.rheuma21st.com/archives/ACR99.html. p 12–13, 1999.

14. Angell M. Is academic medicine for sale? New Engl J Med 2000;342:1516–1518.

15. Kassirer JP. Financial indigestion. JAMA 2000;284:2156–2157.

16. Korn D. Conflicts of interest in biomedical research. JAMA 2000;284:2234–2236.

17. DeAngelis CD. Conflict of interest and the public trust. JAMA 2000;284:2237–2238.

18. Dana J, Loewenstein G. A social science perspective on gifts to physicians from industry JAMA 2003;290:252–255.

19. British Medical Journal. May 31, 2003 (theme issue: "Time to untangle doctors from drug companies").

20. Relman A. Your doctor's drug problem. New York Times, Nov 18, 2003,op-ed page.

21. Association of American Medical Colleges. Industry Funding of Medical Education. Report of an AAMC Task Force. Association of American Medical Colleges, Washington, DC, June 2008. (Available at https://services.aamc.org/Publications/index.cfm?fuseaction=Product.displayForm&prd_id=232&prv_id=281.

22. Matteson E, Panush RS. Eponyms should be abandoned. Rheumatology News 2007;6:12.

23. Matteson E, Panush RS. Eponyms should be abandoned. Reply. Rheumatology News, 2008;7:12.

24. Panush RS. Upon finding a Nazi anatomy atlas: The lessons of Nazi medicine. The Pharos 1996;59:18–22.

25. Panush RS, Paraschiv D, Dorff EN. The tainted legacy of Hans Reiter. Seminars Arthritis Rheum 2003;32:231–236.

26. Panush RS, Wallace DJ, Dorff EN, Engleman EP. Retraction of the suggestion to use the term "Reiter's syndrome" 64 years later: the legacy of Reiter, a war criminal, should not be eponymic honor but rather condemnation. Arthritis Rheum 2007;56:693–694.

27. Panush RS, Sergent JS. A rude awakening. JAMA 1997;277:515–516.

28. Panush RS, Kaplan H. Who will care for our patients? J Rheumatol, 1995;22:2197–2198.

# Chapter 31

# *The Future of Rheumatology*

Edward D. Harris, Jr.

*Alpha Omega Alpha, Menlo Park, CA*

As long ago as the mid-20th century, leaders of rheumatology, both in the United States and abroad, began to realize that this subspecialty of internal medicine had the potential perhaps more than any other—of developing effective therapies for rheumatic diseases directly from discoveries within basic science laboratories. Few of us need to be reminded that it was the discovery and effective use of cortisone, and later, its derivatives, that triggered this link of science and practice. Equally important for our patients was the realization that no effective therapies for rheumatic diseases could be discovered without the basic research that delineated the pathophysiology of these diseases. Classic examples of this include sorting out the metabolism of purines that leads to formation of uric acid, that the glomerulonephritis of systemic lupus erythematosus is caused by deposition of immune complexes, and that rheumatoid synovitis is driven by certain cytokines. These insights led to the development of the xanthine oxidase inhibitors, the success of glucocorticoids and cyclophosphamide in treatment of systemic lupus erythematosus (SLE) nephritis, and anti-tumor necrosis factor (TNF) antibodies/fusion proteins for therapy of rheumatoid arthritis (RA).

Crucial to evolution of our specialty has been the American College of Rheumatology (ACR). Unlike many specialties that have fragmented societies, one for basic science and others for practitioners, those rheumatologists who are clinicians have

*The ACR at 75: A Diamond Jubilee*

appreciated that they are better practitioners when they understand the basis of science underlying the disease processes that they want to alleviate. Similarly, basic scientists appreciate the challenges before them when they observe the complex manifestations of diseases that clinicians face every day. The ACR annual meeting is characterized by clinicians attending reviews of basic science and clinical investigators listening intently to clinical discussions. This assimilation must continue.

## 31.1   WHAT WILL THE FUTURE HOLD FOR RHEUMATOLOGY?

### 31.1.1   Clinical Practice

There is little likelihood that rheumatologists will develop substantial new technology that will generate facile entry to higher tax brackets. Indeed, with the limits placed on reimbursement that are inevitable with the high percentage of gross domestic product (GDP) being consumed by health care, it will be crucial for survival of the specialty that rheumatologists will be creatively efficient. Models of practice will include the following:

(a) Multispecialty groups. The most beneficial of these will be one or two rheumatologists joining a larger group of orthopedic surgeons/physical therapists with particular interests in arthritis and sports medicine. Other options will be large aggregates of physicians, such as Kaiser Permanente. In both contexts, reimbursement will be by fixed (negotiated) salary, with potential for performance bonuses.

(b) Group practice in academia. Those who teach, do clinical research, and develop clinical practices within rheumatology divisions in academic medical centers will be the driving forces for the training of fellows, residents, and students. As now, they will be powerful role models, attracting medical residents to apply for rheumatology fellowships. Their knowledge bases will bridge research and clinical practice.

(c) Efficient rheumatology groups using selected nurse practitioners. Based on trust in the knowledge and good judgment of these allied health practitioners, one rheumatologist can amplify her practice many fold, and when in a group of other rheumatologists, she can minimize night/weekend call.

(d) Boutique practices. This type of practice, with a cadre of patients who prepay for full service by one specialist, has the potential for extending beyond serving only high-income patients. With appropriate legislation, medicare patients could be eligible to join such practices that could provide excellent care with a reasonable reimbursement to the physician without excessively high costs to the consumers.

(e) Micropractices. This type of practice is for one physician, probably using her home as an office, and scheduling appointments by the Internet and voice mail. No nurse or secretary would be used. Billing could be outsourced. Overhead, therefore, will be minimal, but volume and total revenue small as well.

## 31.1.2  Training

The exciting science that supports rheumatology will continue to attract inquisitive and talented young scientists: MDs, PhDs, and MD/PhDs. As is happening with surgical subspecialties, it is likely that pathways to the internal medicine subspecialties will open earlier, perhaps permitting first-year residents planning for clinical practice, not research, to apply for specialty fellowships that will begin after 2 years of internal medicine training.

The Research and Education Foundation (REF) of the ACR will grow with gifts from many sources to become a dominant source of trainee funding. The REF will amplify support for postfellowship young faculty. The newly minted rheumatologists will quickly develop "subsubspecialties" that include those focusing on bone health.

## 31.1.3  Research

Scientific investigation in the sciences related to rheumatology is burgeoning and will continue to do so. Federal funding for science will, for the next decade at least, not increase at rates needed to sustain the growth rate. An adjunct and collaborative funding source will be industry, the biotech firms in particular. All professional societies, including the ACR, will have developed firm and clear ethical statements/rules that will prevent conflicts of interest and commitment among relationships with industry.

Although basic investigation initially will have no obvious link to diseases, as in the past, the new technology will quickly be applied to solving questions in pathophysiology and treatment. The exponentially rapid development of new technologies for biological research, including highly specialized nanoimaging, will demand of all investigators that they develop collaborative studies with other laboratories doing seemingly unrelated research, but that, in fact, are essential for completing answers to the questions that they are seeking to solve.

*31.1.3.1  Personalized Medicine.*  Within the next decade, and certainly before the 100th anniversary of the ACR, the DNA sequences of vast numbers of individuals will be recorded on microchips and available for multiple purposes. The genetic variations among individuals will be found to determine the person's susceptibility to disease as well as the probability of his or her responding to certain therapies or developing allergies to specific drugs, many of which we have in our therapeutic arsenals now [1]. Knowing who will respond to therapy with minimal risk of toxicity that affects other cohorts will literally amplify the effectiveness of currently used medications, including the biologic compounds.

*31.1.3.2  Disease Focused Research.*  Within the past several years, rheumatoid arthritis has become the poster child for targeted therapy [2], and the techniques used for RA are being mimicked for sorting out new therapeutic options for other inflammatory musculoskeletal diseases, particularly systemic lupus erythematosus, polymyositis/dermatomyositis, scleroderma, and the various forms of vasculitis. Among these targets are the following:

- Transcription factors
- Antisense nucleotides
- Protein kinases
- Cytokine/chemokine receptors
- Metalloproteases
- Regulators of cell life
- Costimulatory molecules

Initial success with infliximab and etanercept has been followed by three additional anti-TNF antibodies, and additional ones directed are ripe for development for RA therapy are gene therapy and stem cell therapy.

**31.1.3.3   *Gene Therapy.*** Because inflamed joints can be approached directly, the strategy of intraarticular gene therapy is a logical one [3]. Vectors to carry genes into patients' cells will be developed that are nonpathogenic in humans, can transduce both dividing and nondividing cells, and do not integrate into target cell genomes. Adeno-associated virus 5 (AAV), which is a small single-stranded parvovirus that can transduce many cell types is a particularly good candidate. As with almost all novel therapies, exhaustive research using small animals will be essential to establish both proof of concept and effectiveness/safety.

**31.1.3.4   *Stem Cell Therapy.*** Whereas current emphasis is primarily on hematopoietic stem cells (HSCs) generated without ever having to create or destroy an embryo, these induced pluripotent stem (iPS) cells will be transformed into all types of specialized cells. Research will also focus on mesenchymal stem cells (MSCs) that can differentiate into osteocytes, chondrocytes, and smooth-muscle cells [4]. In addition, the MSCs have (in animal cell cultures and in vivo) have suppressive activity on lymphocyte proliferation, perhaps by shifting from a Thelper1 (Th1) to a Th2 dominant population. HSC therapy will require immune system ablation and reconstitution. An integral component of this strategy is building extensive databases that list the genetic characteristics of every potential patient. Already in progress in both Europe and the United States is a comparison of autologous HSC transplantation and intravenous pulse cyclophosphamide in the treatment of patients with severe progressive systemic sclerosis [5].

**31.1.3.5   *Vaccines.*** This strategy is similar to what is already the basis for childhood vaccination: inducing a B-cell response that will generate an autoantibody against the target molecule. Molecular science will produce immunogens that combine peptides of target molecules, virus particles, T-cell epitopes, and glycosaminoglycans [6]. This technology will be particularly useful for SLE and the multiple forms of vasculitis, providing alternatives to glucocorticoid and cyclophosphamide therapy.

**31.1.3.6    *The Future.*** It is impossible to predict with accuracy, and therefore any predictions will be argued by others who have equal insight into what has not happened. What can be used, however, is trajectory, and the path of rheumatology is accelerating. Clinical and investigative rheumatology are on a parallel course, generating an exciting profession for trainees and, most important, better lives— more free of morbidity and premature mortality—for our patients.

## REFERENCES

1. Crow MK. Collaboration, genetic associations, and lupus erythematosus. N Engl J Med 2008;358:956–961.

2. Magrey MN. Treatment of rheumatic diseases in the future: Novel strategies Rheumatol Rep 2008;59–65.

3. Vervoordeldonk MJ, Tak PP. Gene therapy in rheumatic diseases. Best Pract Res Clin Rheumatol 2001;15:771–788

4. Le Blanc K, Frassoni F, Ball L, et al. Mesenchymal stem cells for treatment of steroid-resistant, severe, acute graft-versus-host disease: a phase II study. Developmental Committee of the European Group for Blood and Marrow Transplantation. Lancet 2008; 371:1579–1586.

5. Farge D, Passweg J, van Laar JM, et al. Autologous stem cell transplantation in the treatment of systemic sclerosis: report from the EBMT/EULAR Registry. Ann Rheum Dis 2004;63:974–981.

6. Zagury D, Burny A, Gallo RC. Toward a new generation of vaccines: the anti-cytokine therapeutic vaccines. Proc Natl Acad Sci USA 2001;98:8024 8029.

# Index